INTRODUCTION TO
CLINICAL NEUROLOGY

INTRODUCTION TO

Clinical Neurology

SIR GORDON HOLMES
M.D., F.R.S.

Revised by
BRYAN MATTHEWS
D.M., F.R.C.P.

THIRD EDITION

E. & S. LIVINGSTONE LTD.
EDINBURGH AND LONDON
1968

First Edition	.	.	*1946*
Reprint	.	.	*1947*
Second Edition	.	.	*1952*
Reprint	.	.	*1960*
Third Edition	.	.	*1968*

SBN 443 00231 2

PRINTED IN GREAT BRITAIN

Preface to the Third Edition

WHETHER or not he has read the "Introduction to Clinical Neurology" every physician who conducts an informed examination of the nervous system owes something to the teaching of the late Sir Gordon Holmes. It was with some trepidation, therefore, that I approached the task of revision of the classic text. Major alterations have been concerned with changing concepts of muscular tone and an approach to epilepsy less closely linked to the original observations of local cortical function. A short section on neurology in infancy also seemed appropriate. It proved impossible to evade all temptation to effect minor alterations and additions reflecting my own views, and the need for clarity has imposed a few changes in the author's highly individual style.

A text on neurology containing no mention of treatment and little description of specific diseases might be thought to be of doubtful value. Sir Gordon Holmes' stated aim was, however, to encourage "an intelligent approach to neurology" and such encouragement cannot be judged entirely superfluous today. I have therefore adhered to his scheme of interpreting signs and symptoms as far as possible in terms of disordered anatomy and physiology.

BRYAN MATTHEWS

1968

Preface to the First Edition

THIS book does not pretend to be more than its title implies, an introduction to the study of disorders of the nervous system. It is not its aim to describe or deal with injuries and diseases as such, but to discuss the nature and the significance of the symptoms and abnormal signs which a patient with a nervous disorder may present or which may be revealed by clinical examination. It is based on the experience of teaching during several years in the National Hospital for Nervous Diseases, and has been written in the hope that it may not only prove useful to students, but also recall to some of my former helpers and to visitors to the wards our clinical rounds and discussions.

An intelligent approach to the study of neurology demands some knowledge of the anatomy and physiology of the nervous system, for without this the student cannot hope to attain an adequate understanding of the disturbances of function that constitute symptoms, or employ them in rational diagnosis and treatment. Although it is assumed he is already familiar with its structure and with the basic principles of neurophysiology, a short review of the anatomy and of the functions of each system is included in the chapter in which its disorders are discussed. Where, as in many instances, the exact nature of function has not yet been finally elucidated, or where conflicting views are held, the hypothesis that seems most probable, or that which serves best to explain the symptoms of its disease, is presented. Though to-morrow may disprove some of them, they are put forward in the belief that "truth comes more readily from error than from confusion."

Ancillary methods in diagnosis, as examination of the cerebrospinal fluid, the use of X-rays, ventriculography and electro-encephalography, are not dealt with. No one can doubt their importance, but a clinical study of each patient should always precede their use, for the information they provide can be properly assessed only by the clinician who is fully acquainted with the nature and the location of the disease of the patient.

Technical and ambiguous terms have been avoided as far as possible, and the illustrations which have been selected to supplement the text are mainly simple diagrams.

With rare exceptions authorities are not cited and no references are given, as it is expected that to the student whose interest is excited larger textbooks will be available.

GORDON HOLMES

LONDON,
March, 1946

Contents

Chapter I

Symptoms and Signs

THE diagnosis of pathological conditions in the nervous system implies the determination of the site of the disease, the recognition of the manner in which the pathological process disorders function, and the nature of the pathological lesion.

Localisation is a matter of stating in terms of anatomy the parts or structures involved, and therefore requires a knowledge of anatomy; determination of the manner in which functions are disordered naturally necessitates an acquaintance with the physiology or functions of the diseased organ, and recognition of the nature of the lesion depends on knowledge of the morbid factors which may involve the nervous system and the mode of its reaction to them.

In the nervous system accurate localisation of pathological conditions and recognition of their mode of action are more easily possible than in most other organs. They depend on careful observation of the symptoms and physical signs presented by the patient, and interpretation of the facts observed by the aid of physiology and anatomy. The nature of the lesion, however, can be inferred only from the nature of the symptoms and the order and manner in which they appeared, supplemented by collateral clinical, pathological or other evidence after it has been sorted out and evaluated by the experience of the clinician. The final diagnosis is often as dependent on an accurate history as on a clinical examination.

The distinction between *symptoms*, that is disorders described by the patient, and *physical signs* or the deviations from the normal revealed by examination, while usually sufficiently obvious, cannot be absolute. Pain, for instance, can only be a symptom and yet the reaction to pain is a physical sign. Many important physical signs, such as reflex changes, do not directly disturb the patient but for descriptive purposes it is often convenient to refer to such abnormalities as *symptoms* of nervous disease. Both symptoms and signs must be, in the first place, interpreted as disturbances of normal function which may or may not be due to structural disease, and only later correlated with an anatomical lesion, if such be present. The paresis of voluntary movement in hemiplegia, for example, should be looked upon as the result of failure of conduction of certain impulses through corticospinal neurons and not immediately described in terms of an anatomical lesion, as a softening or hæmorrhage in the internal capsule which interrupts the passage of these impulses.

The first essential, therefore, in intelligent diagnosis is to attempt to interpret symptoms and physical signs in terms of disordered function, and not to treat them as mere clues which, with the aid of an index or key, may point to the nature and site of the disease.

The relation of symptoms to anatomical lesions varies at different levels of the nervous system. The lower levels are more highly organised in the sense that there is here a "high degree of perfection of union and certainty of action of nervous elements with one another" (Hughlings Jackson). Their functions are consequently more rigid, more sharply restricted and less modifiable than many of those of higher levels, and there is less possibility of the activity of other parts compensating or replacing their functions when these are lost or impaired. When a peripheral nerve is divided and the rest of the nervous system is thereby cut off from the periphery where the muscles and sensory nerve endings, which are its essential tools, are situated, the relation is most direct; the disturbance of function corresponds closely to the site and severity of the injury.

But even here the loss of function may be to some extent replaced, as by the overlapping of sensory fibres from adjacent nerves, or by the use of muscles innervated by an unaffected nerve. The various "trick movements" or devices by which a patient with a local muscular palsy overcomes his difficulties, as grasping an object between thumb and index by flexion of the thumb when the adductor and opponens of the thumb are weak, or avoidance of double vision due to palsy of an ocular muscle by tilting the head so that contraction of the weak muscle is not required in directing the eyes on the object the patient wishes to inspect, may obscure the total loss of power which exists.

The relation of disturbances of function to structural disease is less close when symptoms are caused by damage of conducting tracts and subcortical masses of grey matter within the central nervous system, as here there is greater opportunity for other systems to substitute, to some extent at least, the functions which are impaired or lost.

In the cortex of the forebrain the relation of function to local structure is more variable. Certain functions are rigidly localised in highly specialised centres, and destruction of such a centre may abolish permanently the function represented in it. This holds mainly for the receptive areas through which the cortex receives impressions from the inner and outer world. It is particularly the case in the visual cortex, a minute lesion of which may cause irreparable loss in a portion of the fields of vision. Localisation is less discrete and rigid in cortical areas through which the brain initiates movement and other reactions; injury of a small portion of the so-called motor cortex may produce little or no permanent disability. But here a distinction must be made between various categories of movement, as those which have been learned or acquired by experience are more dependent on integrity of the cortex, and consequently suffer most regularly and severely when it is damaged.

Complicated and highly integrated actions and forms of behaviour are not represented as such in the forebrain; only their components depend on local areas, and though certain of these only are lost, their loss may disorganise or impair correct performance of the act as a whole. The symptoms of the disease of the forebrain are consequently less regular and stereotyped, and there is, as a rule, a less close correlation between them and the structural lesions to which they are due, than is found in affections of lower levels of the nervous system.

But the student of clinical phenomena must always bear in mind that in the nervous system, and particularly in its higher levels, the localisation of symptoms and the localisation of function are not identical problems. Failure to recognise this distinction has often led to the error of supposing the function of the brain or any part of it to be the prevention of symptoms.

The interpretation of symptoms is often complicated by the remarkable capacity of the nervous system of adapting itself to changed conditions imposed on it by disease. Even when a flexor muscle is grafted to the tendon of an extensor muscle it may give up its lifelong habit of flexing a joint and learn to extend it; and when the proximal end of one nerve is sutured to the distal portion of another of different function it may, when regenerated, serve to innervate an entirely new set of peripheral organs. Similarly, when I reverse the position of the pen in my hand I can, without hesitation, continue to write accurately with the dorsum of my hand towards the paper, though many of the movements employed are the reverse of those I normally use.

Any unnatural or abnormal mode of performance is, however, a pathological symptom even though the act is carried out efficiently. The essential point is not whether the act is possible, but the manner in which it is done. Even though its execution may be correct and adequate to its purpose its performance may be slower, less immediate and precise, or it may require more effort.

A distinction can be drawn between *primary* symptoms directly due to loss of function and *secondary* symptoms due either to attempts to perform a desired act by other means, or to adjustment of the organism to new conditions. The practical importance of such a classification is, however, limited as it is clearly difficult to determine to what extent a clumsy movement is due to loss of function or to inefficiency of surviving nervous structures.

As will be emphasised later, more can often be learned of a patient's disabilities by observing his ordinary actions, as dressing or undressing, walking when apparently unobserved, and his use of tools, as a pen, scissors or a knife and fork, than by specific tests, though these usually permit a more complete analysis of symptoms. Such observations reveal the appropriateness, the rate, the amount and the harmony of movement, defects of which may be less apparent when attention is keyed up during the performance of special tests.

NATURE OF SYMPTOMS

Most anatomical lesions are destructive, and consequently abolish or impair the normal activity of the parts they involve. It is obvious that such destructive or negative lesions can cause directly only *negative symptoms*, that is, loss or defect of function. The immediate result of injury of the motor cortex or of the cerebrospinal tract, for instance, is paralysis or feebleness of certain movements of the opposite limbs.

But *positive symptoms*, or manifestations of excess of functional activity, often accompany them. Removal of a cat's forebrain produces decerebrate rigidity or increase of tone in certain groups of muscles, and hemiplegic limbs become hypertonic and their reflexes are exaggerated. The usual interpretation of such positive symptoms is that they are due to over-activity of levels or physiological mechanisms which normally are inhibited or kept under control by a part that is damaged. They are "released," and consequently react excessively to stimuli which come either from without or originate within the body.

But release from control or lack of inhibition does not account for all the symptoms which can be looked upon as positive and interpreted as due to over-activity of intact structures, for when a complex mechanism is disturbed there may be a reorganisation of function in related parts which modifies the clinical picture that might be expected to result from a simple destructive lesion.

The three main factors in the production of symptoms in the presence of a destructive lesion of the nervous system are, therefore: (1) negative symptoms which are a direct result of the injury; (2) positive symptoms due to release of related or subordinate parts; (3) reorganisation or modification of functions of uninjured physiological mechanisms.

Positive symptoms are, however, occasionally due to lesions which "irritate" or excite the activity of nervous elements, particularly those contained in grey matter of the central nervous system, as the spasms or convulsions often associated with disease of the motor cortex. A feature of these symptoms is that they are intermittent or spasmodic; persisting disturbances of function of any part of the central nervous system are rarely, if ever, due to "irritation." In the peripheral nervous system, on the other hand, positive symptoms are not uncommonly due to irritative lesions, as the pain associated with compression or inflammation of sensory nerve fibres, or the spasm of one side of the face which sometimes follows injury of the facial nerve.

Abnormalities of function, whether regarded as symptoms or physical signs, can therefore be classified as:

(1) *Primary or direct*, that is, immediately due to the lesion. The majority are *negative*, that is, they indicate loss or reduction of function since most lesions are destructive. But *positive* symptoms occasionally occur, as pain associated with injury of a peripheral nerve, and spasms and

convulsions with disease of the grey matter of the central nervous system.

(2) *Secondary or indirect* disorders, which are usually *positive*, that is, they indicate over-activity of certain nervous mechanisms owing to—

(*a*) Release from inhibition normally exerted by the injured parts:

or (*b*) Disordered reactions, or disintegration of function of physiological mechanisms of which part had been injured.

CHAPTER II

Pathology

THE morbid anatomy of various affections of the nervous system does not come within the intention of this book. By pathology is meant the manner in which anatomical lesions disorder function. In this sense it is morbid physiology. It is therefore necessary to understand how different forms of disease may influence or disturb physiological activity before an attempt can be made to correlate symptoms with anatomical lesions.

Diseases of the nervous system can be classified as *local lesions* which are limited to one region and injure all the tissues within it regardless of their structures or functions; *diffuse disease*, consisting essentially of multiple local lesions, in which the damage of functional elements is frequently incomplete and certain nerve cells and fibres suffer more severely than others; and *systemic or parenchymatous affections* in which anatomically and functionally related systems of cells or fibres are predominantly involved.

Damage or destruction of nervous elements by *local lesions* is usually secondary to pathological processes that in the first place affect other tissues. It may be a patch of inflammation in which the vascular and supporting tissues are primarily involved and the nerve cells and fibres suffer as a result; a hæmorrhage which breaks up the tissue; a necrosis due to vascular occlusion; a tumour which either invades or compresses the part, or a trauma which damages it. Such a lesion may be complete and destroy all the nervous structures within its limits, or partial, in which case it produces symptoms by disturbing, but not destroying, the anatomical integrity, and, therefore, the functional capacity, of cells and fibres, or by involving a certain number of them only. Certain neurotropic viruses, however, as those of poliomyelitis and rabies, attack nerve cells directly; the accompanying vascular reactions, cellular infiltration and proliferation of neuroglia are secondary.

Though fibres of peripheral nerves which have been divided can regenerate and regain their function, in the central nervous system complete destructive lesions cause irreparable damage, since fibres which have been interrupted and cells which have been severely injured never recover. Some recovery may, however, occur for other parts, or other nervous mechanisms may compensate or replace, though to a limited extent only, the functions of the tissues which are destroyed. Such compensation is more likely when the lesion involves higher levels of the nervous system, as the forebrain, for though function is here more specialised it is less organised and may be less exclusively localised than in lower levels.

The amount of functional disturbance which results from a less severe or partial lesion depends on the stage of the disease, on its mode of onset and on the parts involved in it. When a lesion develops suddenly or rapidly negative symptoms are always greater and usually more widespread immediately after its onset. This is due partly to recovery, after a period of days or weeks, of cells and fibres which were not seriously damaged, and partly to the fact that acute lesions are frequently surrounded by zones of œdema and circulatory changes which produce more extensive disorders of function. Swelling of the affected tissues may also compress neighbouring structures.

Slowly progressive lesions, on the other hand, usually cause less severe disturbances in relation to their extent and severity. The symptoms that result from compression of the spinal cord or of the cortex by a slowly growing tumour, for instance, are always less pronounced than those due to trauma or rapid compression causing anatomical changes of comparable severity.

But another important factor in the production of symptoms by acute lesions is *shock* or temporary depression of function. Shock may be local, that is, restricted to the tissues involved in, but not destroyed by, the lesion and to those in its immediate neighbourhood, but the functional activity of more distant but anatomically and physiologically related parts may also be depressed. For instance, when the spinal cord is suddenly cut across or severely injured, the tone of the muscles and the reflexes of the lower limbs, which depend on the isolated but anatomically intact segments, disappear for a time. Similarly, in a case of acute hemiplegia due to a vascular accident in the forebrain muscle tone and the reflexes in the paralysed limbs may be absent for days; the sudden interruption of the pyramidal tract, or rather loss of impulses carried by it and other descending fibres to the spinal centres that innervate the palsied limbs, depresses temporarily their functional activity. In the same way an acute lesion of the sensory cortex may reduce or abolish sensibility to pain by the effect of shock on subcortical centres. It was to this distant shock or depression of function that von Monakow applied the term "diaschisis."

As cells and fibres which were damaged but not destroyed by an incomplete acute lesion recover gradually, as œdema and other changes around it subside, and as the effects of shock pass off, the intensity of the symptoms diminishes and the final state depends wholly on the severity of the injury and on the structures involved in it.

Symptoms which accompany local lesions also depend to some extent on the relative vulnerability of cells and fibres to the pathological agents to which they are subjected. The cells of the grey matter suffer more quickly from failure of blood supply than the fibres of the white matter. Even the susceptibility of different groups of cells to anoxæmia and other pathological agents varies; the cortical pyramids, for example, degenerate more rapidly than the motor cells of the anterior horns of the cord when their blood supply is cut off. On the other hand, a patch of disseminated sclerosis which extends over both grey and white matter interferes more seriously with the functions of the latter. When a mixed nerve is compressed conduction through the motor fibres is usually interrupted before conduction through the sensory fibres, and pressure upon the spinal cord may block conduction through certain tracts more severely than that through others.

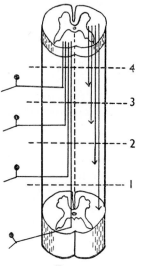

FIG. 1.

Diagram to represent the effect of four incomplete lesions of the spinal cord. If it is assumed that all the lesions are of equal intensity it is evident that the longest ascending and descending fibres are subjected to four times as great injury as the shortest.

Diffuse Disease.—These diseases are characterised by scattered or multiple lesions which usually occur in irregular succession, widely distributed throughout the nervous system but with relative predilection for specific regions according to the nature of the pathological process.

Occlusive vascular disease, disseminated sclerosis and meningo-vascular syphilis, for example, all present special features, but their symptoms differ in no essential manner from those caused by local or circumscribed lesions. The same factors determine the nature and the course of the symptoms. Apart from the distribution, severity and extent of the pathological process they depend on its mode of onset, its rate of development and on the vulnerability of different elements of the tissue to it. The tendency of longer fibres to suffer more severely than those of a shorter course can be explained by the fact that they are involved by several patches of disease, each of which adds its quota to the total damage, while shorter fibres may escape or may be damaged by one or two foci only (Fig. 1).

Another factor which determines symptoms in disease that does not destroy the tissues it involves is the tendency for the more specialised and more highly evolved functions to suffer first and most severely. This is the principle emphasised by Hughlings Jackson as *dissolution*, that is, in disease functions tend to suffer in the reverse order to their appearance in the course of evolution. The newer anatomical structures and the more highly differentiated functions are more severely affected. The law of dissolution consequently applies to the forebrain.

Systemic Disease.—Many diseases of the nervous system of unknown cause are characterised by symptoms and signs suggesting predominant or exclusive involvement of certain functionally related systems of cells or fibres. Pathological examination does not, however, confirm that, for example, the degeneration in Friedreich's ataxia is limited to the pyramidal and spino-cerebellar tracts, or that motor neurons alone are involved in motor neuron disease, but the concept of systemic disease is still useful. The same pattern is observed in many biochemical lesions of the nervous system in which the cause is at least partially understood. Thus in the inborn error of metabolism, Wilson's disease, the lenticular nucleus is predominantly affected, although there are also widespread unsystematised lesions. Deficiency of vitamin B_{12} causes degeneration of the spinal pyramidal tracts and posterior columns but also diffuse cerebral symptoms. External toxins may show similar partial selectivity. The lesions of carbon monoxide poisoning commonly predominate in the pallidum while thalidomide caused peripheral axonal degeneration, apparently mainly in afferent fibres.

The relationship of systemic disease as here defined to known biochemical, toxic and nutritional causes suggests that similar factors may be operative in those systemic degenerations of unknown cause. In general such diseases are symmetrical in their impact on the nervous system and progressive, but there are numerous exceptions.

CHAPTER III

Examination of the Patient

THERE is perhaps no branch in practical medicine in which the help and co-operation of the patient is so essential as in the approach to a neurological disorder. For, in the first place, it is on the patient we must mainly rely for an accurate history of the development of his illness, and such a history is often extremely valuable in determining its nature. Loss of power of movement or of sensation in the legs, for example, may be due to a traumatic injury of the cord, to a meningo-myelitis, or to compression, and the symptoms produced by these three causes may be more or less identical; but a history of a sudden onset points to the first, a sub-acute onset to the second, while a slow and gradual development of the disability is more probably due to spinal compression.

In the second place, many neurological symptoms are purely subjective; they are abnormalities experienced by the patient, and may be accompanied by no outward or visible sign of disease. It is consequently only by his descriptions of them that we can learn anything of their nature and distribution.

Finally, in the examination of the functions of the special senses and of sensibility we must rely on the patient's co-operation, as it is only from information he conveys to us that we can learn if the stimuli we employ evoke normal sensations.

The attitude of the patient to the examination is, therefore, of prime importance, and the first duty of the observer is to obtain his co-operation and interest. A detached or disinterested approach often fails to do so. When the problem is diagnosis of a disability of which the patient complains, it should be explained to him that a thorough investigation, and one not merely restricted to the part to which he refers his symptoms, may be necessary to determine its nature before steps can be taken to remove or relieve it.

Most neurologists adopt a comprehensive scheme for the examination of the functions of the nervous system, and there can be no doubt that such a scheme is essential to assure complete and methodical investigation, but it must be remembered that the patient's interest is focused on his main symptom, and that it may flag if this is not dealt with early. He may, for instance, fail to understand the value or significance of starting with an ophthalmoscopic examination, or of testing the pupillary reflexes, when his main trouble is weakness of a leg. Any scheme employed should therefore be elastic, and the order of tests should be varied according to the circumstances of each case.

When the investigation is necessarily long, and when its purpose is not immediately apparent to the patient his interest should be stimulated by any means possible. This can often be done by explaining the results of the tests which are employed, or by encouraging competition with previous results or those obtained on examination of another part.

The *history of the illness* should be, in the first place, obtained and recorded as far as possible in the patient's own words: the observer should intervene as little as possible, and only to exclude obviously irrelevant matter, to obtain amplification on statements which are vague or seem incomplete, or to lead his story into directions in which useful information may be obtained. It is often advisable to point out to the patient that it is facts, not his interpretation of them, which are required, for both educated and uneducated patients, and particularly the former, often prefer to give their own views on the diagnosis and causation of their disabilities than to describe them.

It is also essential to ascertain the exact meaning attached by the patient to the words and terms he employs. Language often fails to provide unambiguous terms for many common subjective symptoms, for they are outside the range of normal experience, and the same term may be applied to symptoms which are essentially different. Loss of sensation in a hand, a purely negative phenomenon, may be described as numbness, and the same word may be used for the sensation associated with a local epileptic attack, where it is a positive disturbance, that is, something added to the normal sensibility of the part. Similarly, the term "giddiness" may be used to describe an attack of vertigo, lack of balance, or merely a dazed feeling or a feeling of faintness. It is only by persistent questioning that the observer can learn the nature of the disorder of which the patient speaks.

As the patient's attention is usually focused on the symptom or symptoms which appear to him the most important, he may fail to mention others which are equally significant, and it must always be borne in mind that the absence of certain symptoms is often as important as their presence. Consequently, when he has given his own story it is usually necessary to supplement it by questions, but as patients are often suggestible and readily accept any suggestions offered by the examiner, these questions should be, in the first place, indirect. If, for example, it is desired to learn if he has had diplopia, he should be asked if his sight had ever been disturbed, and only if he replies "no" should he be asked directly if he has seen double. Similarly, if there is the history of an attack which may have been epileptic, it is advisable to enquire if after he had recovered he noticed anything wrong in his mouth or with his clothes, rather than in the first place to enquire if he had bitten his tongue or passed urine.

The sequence of events in the evolution of an illness often throws valuable light on its nature. It is, therefore, important to obtain a history of the onset of each symptom and learn whether it has been constant or intermittent, has advanced regularly or been stationary. For this purpose one of two methods can be adopted. The patient may either describe his condition week by week or month by month since his illness commenced, stating when each new symptom appeared or how those already present had altered: in other words, he gives a chronological story of his illness. But it is often more satisfactory to deal with the history of each symptom separately, and then combine them into a consecutive story.

The history of an illness thus obtained from the patient, supplemented by facts gleaned by indirect or direct questioning, frequently fails to give a concise or complete picture of its development. It is therefore often advisable for the examiner to reconstruct it, and record it as concisely and in as simple words as possible. It may then be read or presented to the patient to be corrected or confirmed by him.

It is usually necessary to complete the history by specific questions, particularly when symptoms are wholly subjective. Whether it be disturbance of movement, pain, numbness, tingling or other sensory disturbance, even headache, it is advisable to follow a definite system of investigation. A satisfactory method is to determine: (a) the exact nature of each symptom; (b) its relations in space; (c) its relations in time; (d) the factors which influence it.

For instance, the patient should in the first place describe, as far as words serve him, the exact nature of each symptom; then indicate its distribution or the area over which it extends; say whether it is constant, and if not constant its frequency, the hours of the day and the circumstances under which it occurs; and, finally, what may excite it, aggravate it or relieve it.

It is often necessary and sometimes essential, to supplement the history obtained from the patient by independent testimony, for an observer can often give more useful information, and may add important facts neglected or forgotten by him. This is frequently the case where there have been disorders of consciousness, conduct or behaviour, or change in the mental state. It is also important to obtain, if possible, independent descriptions of accidents or seizures accompanied by loss or disturbances of consciousness or of memory.

An investigation of the mental state of the patient should be included in the formal examination, but certain facts should be noted while he gives his history. The value of the story he tells can be estimated only when it is ascertained whether his memory is reliable or not. Lack of attention or a tendency to fatigue may have to determine the scope and duration of the examinations which should follow. The patient's attitude to his symptoms and towards his illness is often significant: the anxious, neurotic patient is obsessed with every detail, and constantly adds to or elaborates his story; while the general paralytic may deny he suffers in any way, or may be satisfied to speak of his prominent symptoms only.

The frequent existence of psychogenic disorders, either alone or combined with symptoms of organic disease, in patients who come under his care also makes it essential for the neurologist to consider the individual as a whole; his personality, his reactions and his behaviour are often as valuable indications in diagnosis as the physical signs elicited in examination.

The mode of response to questions and to special tests should be carefully observed, delay or hesitancy in reply, or obvious doubt in the correctness of his response when the strength of the stimulus employed is well above the normal threshold, usually indicates some disorder of function, provided it does not also occur when normal parts are examined.

PHYSICAL EXAMINATION

The adoption of a systematic scheme or method for the examination of neurological cases assures, in the first place, that no important physical sign will be missed, and, in the second place, it enables a complete investigation to be carried out more quickly than if the observer uses haphazard methods. Various such schemes have been recommended, all of which may present some advantages: that described below (p. 181) will be found sufficient for most needs, but it may be necessary to modify it for certain cases.

It is important in conducting such an examination to bear in mind certain facts:

(1) The absence of abnormal physical signs may be just as important as their presence, and must be recorded or noted by the observer. It is usually sufficient to record that no abnormality has been found in, for instance, the motor system, reflexes, sensation, etc.

(2) As is the case in taking the history of the illness, it is often advisable to begin the examination by dealing with the most prominent symptoms, and later to investigate functions apparently unconnected with the patient's complaints.

(3) As the trustworthiness of many observations depends on the subject's co-operation and attention, and as these faculties may give out owing to fatigue or failure of interest, it may be necessary to interpolate in the series of investigations usually adopted, other tests which throw less strain on attention, or in which the patient's co-operation is not so necessary. For example, an investigation of sensation or of the visual fields may be interrupted while the observer examines the heart, the ocular movements or even the motor system.

(4) The significance of slight deviations from the normal may be just as great as that of more pronounced changes; even the slightest may point to important disturbances of function. It is, however, essential that the observer satisfies himself that the deviation is pathological. Failure of a pupil to react briskly to light, or of the toes to flex promptly when the sole of the foot is stimulated, may be as valuable indications of disease as the phenomenon originally described by Argyll Robertson or the form of

plantar reflex known by Babinski's name. Neglect of petty abnormalities and focusing of attention on the existence or absence of certain "signs" is a common cause of errors in diagnosis and of failure to recognise disease. Such "signs" usually develop gradually, and may be just as important when they represent the first deviation from the normal as in their full-blown state. A search for absolute and clear-cut syndromes is foreign to scientific investigation of such biological problems as the physician meets. Though well-known "signs" are often useful for the purpose of description, they should be laid aside or disregarded during the examination of a patient; in this the task of the physician is to determine if there is any disorder of function or abnormality of structure, and then investigate its nature. To describe what is observed merely as this person's or that person's "sign" is often a cloak for a too cursory examination, and when used as an index for the purpose of diagnosis frequently obscures the clinical problem. Further, "signs" often have different meanings to different observers: the term "Argyll Robertson pupil" often signifies merely failure of the reflex contraction to light, and "Babinski's sign" only extensor movement of the great toe, but in their original descriptions each included much more. Even if a too rigid adherence to eponymous signs is avoided descriptions of clinical phenomena frequently become meaninglessly stereotyped. For instance, the word "sluggish" is now almost universally employed to describe reflexes that are reduced in speed or amplitude or both and, by insensible degrees, its use may spread to conceal indecision as to whether the reflex is present at all.

(5) As valuable information is often obtained by observation of the patient's ordinary activities as by specific tests. The manner in which he uses his hands in dressing or undressing himself, in arranging his bedclothes, and even in gestures during conversation, may point to disorders of movement which may be missed in a formal examination. A slight disturbance of gait may be more obvious as the patient approaches us or moves through the room than when he is braced up by the request to show how he çan walk. The attitudes of the patient, his facial expression, his modes of reaction to question or during conversation, may all give valuable clues to the nature of his disabilities. It should not be necessary to emphasise that the patient's specific symptoms must always be investigated. A complaint of difficulty in climbing stairs will seldom be elucidated by examining the patient lying on a couch.

(6) The manner in which a test or action is carried out is often more significant than its performance. The central nervous system has a great capacity of adapting itself to new conditions; if one mode of response is impossible, an alternative method may succeed, but it is an abnormal method, it is a pathological symptom.

(7) Finally, to examine or even to consider the nervous system in isolation is the sign, not of scientific specialisation, but of inferior medicine.

Chapter IV

The Motor Systems

B Y the motor system we move our bodies in space and separate parts of it in relation to one another, and it is also by means of it that we maintain postures and attitudes in opposition to gravity and other external forces.

All movements, apart from those of the visceral organs and of other structures innervated by the autonomic system, are effected by contractions of striated muscles which are initiated and controlled by the nervous system. In man the nervous mechanisms concerned in posture and movement consist of *peripheral or lower motor neurons*, the cells of which lie in the ventral horns of the spinal cord and in corresponding nuclei in the brain-stem, and *suprasegmental centres* in subcortical masses of grey matter and in the cortex of the forebrain and projection fibres that connect these with the lower motor neurons.

The organisation of the lower motor neurons is relatively simple, but that of the central organs of movement is complex and by no means fully elucidated yet. Clinicians distinguish two main systems, the *Cortico-spinal or Pyramidal System*, which consists of a "motor area" in the cortex of each hemisphere and projection fibres which run from it in the pyramidal tract, and an *Extrapyramidal System*, which includes centres in the brain-stem and basal ganglia and efferent fibres from them.

In lower vertebrates, in which the cerebral cortex is rudimentary, all the motor activities of the animal are effected through subcortical centres, but with its greater development in higher mammals some of these functions were transferred to it. The older motor mechanisms in subcortical centres retain, however, many of their original activities, though these have been modified as they came under cortical control; they have not been wholly replaced, but have become incorporated in a more elaborate motor sytem. It is through them that the cortex still carries out many of its reactions; they remain an essential part of the motor machine.

Although for purposes of analysis and description it is convenient to deal with these two motor systems separately, it must not be forgotten that under normal conditions they work together, and that the efficiency of each depends largely on the collaboration of the other.

It is often naively assumed that most of, or even all, our movements are voluntary in the sense that they result directly from an effort of will, but it is evident that there are several classes or varieties of movement, some of which are entirely independent of consciousness, and the degree of consciousness associated with other categories varies.

At one end of the scale are simple reflexes, as the knee-jerk or withdrawal of a foot from a pin-prick. Such reflexes are constant and under stationary conditions invariable, though they may be modified or even suppressed by other reflexes and by the activity of higher levels of the nervous system. More widespread reactions, as those concerned in standing and in righting the body when its equilibrium is threatened, are reflex, too, but they are mediated through supraspinal levels, mainly through the brain-stem.

At the other end of the scale are the more complex, more variable and more flexible or modifiable movements which are initiated by will and accompanied by consciousness: these require control and guidance by mind, and are the elements of deliberate one-at-a-time acts. They are truly voluntary movements. Some are innate but perfected by experience, others are acquired by learning and practice, as those employed in the use of tools. In man these highly differentiated voluntary movements are dependent upon and intimately bound up with the activity of the cerebral cortex, and are readily abolished or impaired by disease of it. Their execution, however, requires the co-operation of subcortical mechanisms the activities of which lie below the verge of consciousness. Even such a simple act as raising an arm necessitates changes in the posture of other parts of the body or alterations in the tension of its muscles; these are brought about by spinal or mesencephalic reflexes.

There are, however, degrees in the voluntary element of movement. Many acts which were originally dependent on the constant guidance of mind become less so when repeatedly performed. Knitting, for instance, is a complicated act which is learned slowly by concentration on individual movements of the fingers, but by practice becomes less conscious: a woman may read or engage in conversation while knitting. The act has become more automatic. Many ordinary activities fall into the same category. A child learns to walk by attention to the necessary movements of his limbs and trunk, but in later life walking is less dependent on conscious control. The pattern of the action, that is the arrangement and synthesis of its constituent movements, is apparently established or laid down in the cortex, and it is from the cortex that the action is initiated. Though sub-cortical mechanisms may take a greater part in the execution of acts which have become automatic their performance is still dependent upon the activity of the cortex, an injury of which may disturb or abolish them.

Other automatic actions, as blinking and swinging the arms while walking, seem to be wholly subserved by subcortical centres. Expressional movements, as smiling, weeping and expressions of anger and pleasure, originate in areas remote from the motor cortex, and may be unimpaired when the corresponding voluntary movement is impossible. When, for instance, one side of the face is paretic as a result of a cortical lesion, it may move as freely as the other when the patient smiles.

Finally, as a link between purely reflex movements subserved by the spinal cord and brain-stem and more highly integrated voluntary and automatic movements, there are a series of reflexes which require the intervention of perception and are dependent on the integrity of portions of the cerebral cortex, as blinking to a flash of light or when an object suddenly approaches the eyes, and movement of the eyes towards a light or an object.

Not only are there many varieties of movement, but the same motor act may belong to different physiological categories; it is only by their origin and purpose they can be classified. For instance, closure of the lids may be automatic, as in ordinary blinking; it may be a reflex excited by a stimulus to the cornea or by a flash of light; or a reflex of higher order, as to the threat of an approaching object; it may be part of an emotional response, as in laughter or crying, or a purely intentional or voluntary act.

While reflex and automatic movements may continue for long periods without tiring, intentional movements when long continued require more and more conscious effort and tire more rapidly. Though we blink automatically and without discomfort through our waking hours, voluntary closure of our lids when repeated for long becomes exhausting. Similarly, we swing our arms unconsciously and without effort as we walk, but one who has lost this automatism finds it difficult to do so for long. It is worthy of note that absence of tiring is also a feature of many pathological involuntary movements which, if executed voluntarily, would soon exhaust the patient.

The progress from simple and restricted, but highly organised, reflex movements, and from the more complex and extensive but more modifiable automatic movements which sufficed for animals lower in the phylogenetic scale to the highly differentiated and specialised movements which are at the service of man, has developed parallel with the evolution of the forebrain. The higher we go in the animal scale the greater is the part played by the cerebral cortex in motor activities till in man locomotion and all purposive activities are dependent on it. This does not mean that in man the older motor mechanisms which proved so efficient in lower forms of life have been discarded and remain rudiments of little or no functional importance. The same spinal, bulbar and mesencephalic reflexes are available for various modes of reaction, but the subcortical ganglia, which were the highest centres of motor integration, have lost much of their earlier importance. They have become subordinate to the newer motor system, but the effects of disease show that they play an essential part even in the motor activities of man. The part many of them take in different types of movement has not been definitely determined, and an exact formulation of their functions in the higher vertebrates is not yet possible.

LOWER MOTOR NEURONS

The structure as well as the functions of striated muscles depends on their connection with the central nervous system by means of the peripheral

C

motor nerves which take origin from the ventral horns of the spinal cord and from homologous cells in the brain-stem. These are collectively known as the *Lower Motor Neurons* and, from the point of view of function, as the *Final Common Path*, as it is through them exclusively that all nervous impulses which can influence striated muscles pass. Injuries of the lower motor neurons affect muscles more or less regardless of their functions; the palsies that result are palsies of muscles or of parts of muscles.

Each motor nerve fibre innervates many muscle fibres, the number varying from approximately 2,000 in the large limb muscles to 100 in the intrinsic muscles of the hand and probably even fewer in the ocular and facial muscles. A single lower motor neuron and the muscle fibres it supplies constitute a "motor unit." The existence in every muscle of separate motor units which can be brought into action singly or in any combination is one of the factors by means of which motor responses can be graded.

The arrangement of the motor cells in the ventral horns was originally metameric, those of one segment innervated the muscles of the corresponding myotome, and though in the human spinal cord the distinction of segments is more or less artificial a metameric arrangement persists. The fibres of each ventral root take origin in the corresponding segment, but as the roots break up and intermingle in the plexuses from which peripheral nerves are formed, each of the latter may contain fibres from several roots. And as most of the larger muscles are derived from two or more myotomes, they are innervated by fibres from two or more segments which may come to them through a single or through several nerves. The distribution of paralysis due to disease of the cells of a ventral horn, or of a ventral root, may consequently differ from that which results from injury of a motor nerve.

As the anatomical integrity of muscles depends on influences transmitted through the motor neurons, when the latter are injured or diseased the fibres of the muscles waste or degenerate and fail to respond to all nervous impulses. The essential features of disease of the lower motor neurons are therefore: (1) Degeneration of muscle fibres supplied by the affected neurons, and consequently diminution in size or atrophy of the muscle. Later an overgrowth of connective tissue may replace the degenerated fibres, and when it shortens contractures and deformities may develop. (2) Loss of all reflexes, including muscle tone, in which the nerve fibres are concerned. (3) Failure of the muscles innervated by the injured fibres to contract to voluntary and other impulses, that is, paralysis of movement.

Injury to the peripheral fibres of the lower motor neurons may result in axonal degeneration, with results resembling those of anterior horn cell destruction, or in conduction block. Here the function of the fibres is interrupted but they remain in anatomical continuity. The two conditions are not immediately distinguishable as both cause paralysis of the muscles supplied by the nerve but the implications are very different as conduction block recovers without residual disability. The detection of denervation due to axonal loss is of considerable importance in the prognosis of peripheral motor nerve lesions. The electrical "reaction of degeneration" is now of historical interest only as it proved totally unreliable except where the answer was already obvious on clinical grounds. Electromyography and the strength/duration curve are far more reliable indications of the presence or absence of anatomical denervation.

THE UPPER MOTOR NEURONS OR THE CORTICOSPINAL MOTOR SYSTEM

The corticospinal motor system, that is the projection fibres which connect the cerebral cortex with the lower motor neurons of the spinal cord, is the chief and, functionally, the most important of the descending tracts concerned in the initiation of movement and control of posture. As they are collected into compact bundles in the pyramids of the medulla they are generally known as the *pyramidal tracts*.

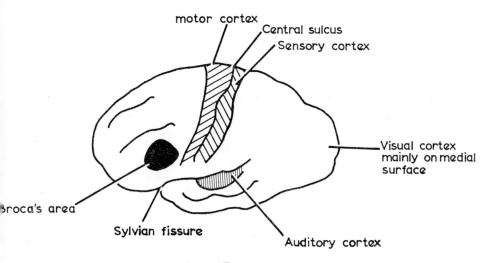

FIG. 2.

The lateral surface of the left hemisphere.

While it is a useful clinical convention to assume that the fibres of the pyramidal tract originate in the excitable precentral motor cortex, (Fig. 2), many fibres arise from cells in the post-central gyrus or in other unknown areas of the brain. These facts, while of undoubted physiological importance, have so far contributed little to the interpretation of the symptoms of disease of the upper motor neuron.

The fibres of the pyramidal tracts which carry impulses spinalwards from the motor area of the cortex pass diffusely through the white matter of the hemispheres, but are collected into compact bundles in the internal capsule and in the peduncles of the mid-brain. They occupy the anterior two-thirds of the posterior limb of the internal capsule; those from the facial centre lie most anteriorly, and then in order those from the hand, arm, shoulder, trunk, thigh, leg and foot areas (Fig. 3). The same order exists in the peduncles, the fibres conveying impulses for facial movements lying most medially, but below this level there is less discrete arrangement of fibres according to their ultimate destination.

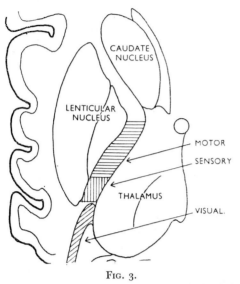

FIG. 3.

Diagram of the internal capsule of the left hemisphere of the brain to show the positions occupied by the motor, sensory and visual projection fibres.

During its course through the brain-stem each pyramidal tract gives off fibres which cross the middle line to the nuclei of the motor cranial nerves of the opposite side. Injury of these fibres after their decussation may rarely cause a supranuclear palsy of certain movements in the head segment, as of the face or tongue, on the side of the lesion, and a similar palsy of the opposite limbs if the pyramidal tract of this side is also involved. *Alternate palsies* are, however, more commonly due to involvement of a motor cranial nerve nucleus or of its root fibres, but this produces a lower motor neuron paralysis accompanied by wasting and loss of tone in the cranial muscles of the same side, and a spastic paresis of the contra-lateral limbs.

At the lower end of the medulla the majority of the fibres of the pyramidal tracts decussate and enter the lateral columns of the opposite sides of the spinal cord, but a certain, though variable, number remain in the same side of the cord (Fig. 4). The function and termination of these uncrossed fibres have not been determined but it is doubtful whether they play any part in the recovery of function in hemiplegia.

Some of the pyramidal fibres terminate in arborisations around the motor cells of the ventral horns, but most end on internuncial cells in the grey matter near the base of the dorsal horns. The latter arrangement facilitates the integration of related impulses of different origin before they reach the lower motor neurons.

The Motor Cortex.—The cortex of the forebrain has been subdivided into a large number of areas each of which is distinguished by the form and arrangement of the nerve cells it contains. Correlation of structure with function is rudimentary but the region in front of the central fissure, or fissure of Rolando, is charac-terised by the presence of large Betz cells in one of its deeper layers and is known as *area* 4, the strip in front of it being *area* 6. As it is from area 4 and the adjoining portion of area 6 that isolated movements of the limbs and trunk can be ob-tained by appropriate stimu-lation this region is generally styled the motor area. Its pos-terior border corresponds to the bottom of the central fissure, in fact a large proportion of it is concealed within the fissure, the front wall of which it covers.

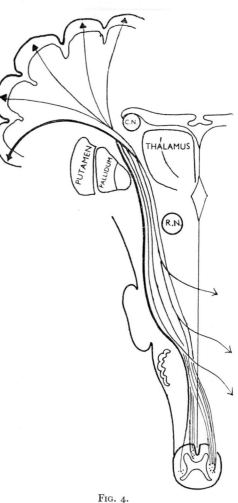

Simple movements and more complex motor reactions can be obtained in both animals and man by electrical stimulation of more extensive regions of the cortex, particularly from more anterior parts of the frontal lobes and from the gyri behind the fissure of Rolando. These may be due to the use of stronger stimuli, to lowering of the thresh-old of excitable points by facili-tation, or to conduction of the stimulus along short association fibres. From the evidence at present available it appears justifiable to restrict the term

Fig. 4.

Diagram of the course of the pyramidal tract.

"motor area" to the cortex on the anterior wall of the central fissure and to the surface of the brain immediately in front of it.

Our knowledge of the functions of the motor cortex is based on experimental stimulation supplemented by analysis of the effects of destructive lesions in animals and man. Such evidence must be crude and fragmentary for the application of electrodes to the exposed cortex can bear but a faint resemblance to physiology and destructive lesions in man are seldom conveniently restricted in size and situation. The findings indicate a localisation of function within the motor cortex in that separate but overlapping areas control movements of different parts of the opposite side of the body. Such movements are said to be "represented" in specific cortical areas but although this word is hallowed by tradition its precise connotations are difficult to define. As will be seen it certainly does not mean that there is an invariable linkage between any given point on the cortex and any specific movement.

One of the most striking features of the cortical motor map is that the areas from which movements of the distal portions of the limbs, that is, of those parts employed in delicate and skilled actions, can be elicited exceeds greatly those from which movements of the trunk and proximal segments of the limbs can be obtained; in fact, the area of cortex is in more or less inverse relationship to the bulk of the muscles involved.

The area of cortex concerned with movements of the eyes and associated movements of the head lie further forward. Their projection fibres pass through the internal capsule anterior to and separate from those of the pyramidal tracts; they may be consequently unaffected by cortical and capsular lesions that cause paralysis of the opposite limbs. Voluntary movements of the eyes may be affected by acute unilateral lesions of these systems but chronic palsies are rare unless there are bilateral lesions.

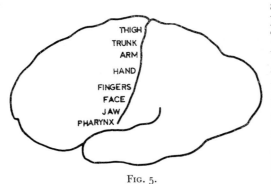

FIG. 5.

Lateral view of the left hemisphere showing the areas of motor cortex from which movement of the different parts of the body can be most easily elicited. The motor cortex concerned with the remainder of the lower limb is on the medial surface.

When stimuli of threshold strength are applied to the cortex only simple or elementary movements, as flexion or extension of a joint, are obtained. Though these primary movements are co-ordinate few of them, when isolated, would serve any specific purpose. Each is only a unit or fraction of a useful action, but each can be variously combined with other units to provide more complete motor reactions. The cortex synthesises them into, or builds up from them, the more complicated actions necessary to or serviceable in ordinary life. As all the words of a language can be represented by combinations of the letters of relatively small alphabets, and as the most complicated music may be produced by the combination and proper arrangement in time of the limited number of notes of a musical instrument, so the cortex can construct from simple components all the movements and actions of which man is, or may ever be, capable.

But the motor cortex cannot be compared with the keyboard of a typewriter or of a musical instrument in which a constant result is obtained

on striking each key. The response of each motor point to adequate stimulation is not fixed or immutable; it may be modified by various factors
and particularly by afferent impulses and by previous activity of itself
or of a neighbouring point. When a response has been evoked it tends
to appear again when adjacent points are stimulated, either in a region
that was previously inexcitable, as in the cortex in front of that which
is generally included in the motor area, or from an adjacent point that
ordinarily yields another movement. Under certain conditions even
an opposite movement may be elicited; if the primary movement was
flexion of a joint it may become extension, or a different, though usually
a related, movement may be obtained. These divergences from the
usual result of stimulation, which are known as facilitation, reversal and
deviation of responses, indicate the functional instability of cortical
motor points and the falsity of any rigid scheme of "representation".

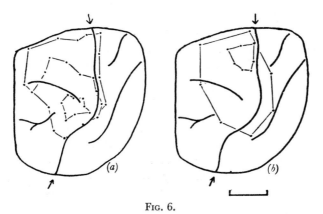

FIG. 6.

The areas of motor cortex of the baboon from which (a) movements
of the thumb and fingers, and (b) of the hallux and middle toe can
be obtained by increasing the strength of the stimulus. Arrows
indicate the central fissure. (Liddell and Phillips.)

The motor cortex must therefore be regarded as a plastic or labile
organ, and it is on this property that its unrivalled power of learning by
education and experience depends. Owing to its functional plasticity a
man, within a few years of his lifetime, may acquire more new and skilled
acts than lower animals, in whom the cortex is less developed, have
succeeded in doing in the course of their whole racial history.

Further, as there is a complete overlap of regions from which movements of different parts of the body can be obtained, even of the fingers
and toes, the so-called motor centres of which are widely separated in the
ordinary cortical map (Fig. 6), it is evident that the functional organisation
of the cortex is more complex than it has been assumed to be. It can no
longer be looked upon as merely an effector mechanism which simply
transmits spinalwards preformed patterns of innervation. Its elaborate

structure and the multiple intracortical communications between its separate points, as well as the innumerable fibres that connect it with other regions of the brain, also indicate it is concerned in the elaboration of impulses that subserve voluntary movement.

Another feature of the cortex is a tendency for strong or prolonged excitation of one of its excitable points to spread to neighbouring points, or even over the whole motor area. This spread usually appears to be from point to point, and it consequently produces a series of movements in a sequence determined by their cortical representation. They are identical with the march of local epilepsy (see p. 136). Sometimes it is less regular or fails to involve a number of intervening points, suggesting that excitation may be conducted by intracortical neurons. When the opposite cortex is involved, as it may be on strong stimulation and in local epilepsy, the spread obviously takes place through commissural fibres.

Its power of initiating and executing fine and skilled voluntary movements makes it necessary that the motor cortex should have lower motor mechanisms under its control; this it does by impulses which may modify or suppress subcortical reactions that would interfere with its own activities, or by breaking them up in order to utilise parts of them for its own purpose, for the forebrain performs its motor acts largely through the agency of subcerebral mechanisms.

The property of building up purposive acts from such small and simple movements as are obtained by stimulation of it does not, however, depend only on the motor area of the cortex. Adjoining portions of the frontal lobes probably play a part in their synthesis, but a stream of impulses from the periphery, many of which never cross the threshold of consciousness, are essential to it. Wider regions of the brain are necessary for the development of complicated actions which require the formulation of an idea of the action intended, and a pattern of its performance. This will be dealt with in the chapter on apraxia (p. 153).

The motor cortex is not, however, an autonomous organ; no part of the brain can function normally when isolated from the rest. The most important influences which act on it are sensory impulses which continually flow to it from various sources. These support or augment its activity; an acute loss of sensation in a limb always causes considerable reduction of power of its voluntary movements and necessitates more effort on the part of the patient. Movements of an anæsthetic limb are also irregular and inco-ordinate; their accuracy, precision and grading are defective owing to faulty arrangement of their components in sequence, range and force. Impressions of proprioceptive origin are in this respect the most important, for apart from the information they provide on the position of the limb at the start of the movement, and of those it occupies in succession during motion, they are necessary for the accurate synthesis of movement and its direction. Other impulses which regulate or modify its activity come from subcortical centres; the cerebellum through its superior peduncle and the thalamus probably exerts an important influence on the motor functions of the cortex. The selection, grading and timing of the components of the motor reaction to the sensory stimuli are normally modified by the factors implicit in the concept of voluntary action.

While the lower motor neurons are concerned in the innervation of individual muscles or parts of muscles, impulses conveyed by the cortico-spinal fibres are concerned with movements only. It is indeed possible to produce movement of single muscles by suitable stimulation of the cortex but the effect of lesions is loss of movements rather than paralysis of muscles. For instance, the long and short extensors of the fingers may be involved separately by injuries of peripheral nerves, but when the functions of either are affected by central disease, those of the other never escape; in other words, the central nervous system is interested only in movement or action, e.g., extension of the fingers, not in the muscles which effect it.

Further, where a muscle may be employed in two separate actions it may fail, owing to a supranuclear lesion, to act in one only: for example, the internal rectus muscle of the eye, which contracts actively in both its lateral deviation to the opposite side and in convergence, may be paralysed in the one movement but normal in the other; and the latissimus dorsi muscle, which takes part in both depression of the arm and in coughing, may be powerless when the former is attempted but normal in the latter action.

Another feature of loss of function of the upper motor neurons is that movements which are habitually bilateral are little affected by lesions of one motor area or of one pyramidal tract. When we frown, or wrinkle our foreheads, or expand our chests voluntarily, as in taking a deep breath, we invariably contract the muscles of both sides of the body concerned in these actions. A one-sided lesion does not paralyse or enfeeble seriously such movements of either side. The usual explanation of this fact is that these movements are normally served by both hemispheres of the brain, and if innervation from one side fails, the other suffices to excite contraction of the muscles on the same as well as of those of the opposite side.

Integrity of the motor cortex is particularly necessary for isolated movements and delicate and finely co-ordinated actions. One of the most striking features of a mild or recovering cortical palsy is inability to flex or extend one finger alone, though the patient can bend or straighten all of them together, or if it is possible the movement is performed slowly and with obvious effort, and lacks precision and delicacy. Similarly, when the cortical centre for movements of one side of the face is injured, he may be unable to wink on this side without at the same time contracting the muscles of his cheek or of the angle of his mouth.

The view often casually accepted that all our motor activities are due exclusively to impulses which are initiated in the cerebral cortex and transmitted to the cord by the pyramidal tracts is certainly incorrect, and presents serious difficulties in the interpretation of clinical symptoms. Though all movements of the body can no doubt be initiated from the cortex it is with the performance of the more voluntary, skilled and learned actions that the cortex is mainly concerned. Less special and more automatic movements, as many of those of the trunk and proximal segments of the limbs, are less exclusively dependent on it, and therefore suffer less when it is damaged; while movements of expression and those which form part of emotional reactions may escape, as they depend on the phylogenetically older structures of the rhinencephalon, though under normal conditions the stimuli which discharge them may originate in the cortex.

The result of extensive damage of the cortical motor area can be seen in an ordinary case of hemiplegia during recovery after the effects of shock have passed off. The finer movements of the fingers and hand are lost, the grosser and less voluntary movements of the proximal segments of the limbs are less affected, the habitually bilateral movements of the trunk and of the upper part of the face are little if at all impaired, and though the voluntary movements of the cheek and lips of the palsied side are reduced in range and power, these parts move as well as those of the opposite side when the patient smiles or weeps.

Some recovery of function is the rule after an acute lesion of the motor cortex, and after removal of a pathological agent, as a tumour. It is partly due to recovery of cells and fibres which were damaged but not destroyed, but this cannot explain it fully. Neighbouring parts of allied function may take on or replace to a very limited extent the functions which were affected; the variability of response of single excitable points to experimental stimuli suggests the possibility that uninjured units may assume functions of those destroyed (Fig. 6). As a certain number of corticospinal fibres pass to the same side of the spinal cord through the direct pyramidal tract, the opposite hemisphere may also substitute that which is injured, but its contribution to recovery of finer movements is doubtful and at most small.

Recovery may be also due to intervention of subcortical structures which normally are engaged in certain categories of movement. There can be little doubt that they take a larger part in so-called voluntary movements than they are generally assumed to do. This is particularly so where a lesion is of long standing, and especially when it developed in early life; the range and power of movement in many cases of infantile hemiplegia, in which the whole motor area and parts of the adjoining cortex are absent or destroyed, is often surprising, but such movements are crude and ill-directed.

In more gradually progressive disease the first sign is usually slowness in the start and awkwardness in the performance of movement, followed by progressive loss of individual movements, those of the distal parts of the limbs being earlier and more severely affected.

Paralysis resulting from lesions limited to the precentral cortex is usually less severe than that due to interruption of the corticospinal pathway in the internal capsule or brain-stem. This may be due to greater destruction of projection fibres where they are collected into compact bundles, but it is probable that movements surviving after cortical lesions are derived partly from more anterior portions of the frontal lobe from which, under experimental conditions, local motor reactions can be elicited (Fig. 6). These are intimately connected with the grey matter of the brain-stem which contains the highest motor mechanisms of lower vertebrates.

During recovery movements of the proximal segments of the limbs are usually regained earlier and more fully than those of the hand and foot. In these it is rarely complete; their movements usually remain slow, require greater effort from the patient, lack natural dexterity and tire easily.

Lost or diminished power of certain movements is the immediate and direct result of destruction of the motor cortex; it is a negative symptom, and only negative symptoms can be directly due to destructive lesions. But positive symptoms, or manifestations of excess of function, also appear after lesions of the upper motor neurons, as exaggeration of the spinal reflexes and increase of muscle tone. These positive symptoms are attributed to absence of inhibitory impulses which permits excessive or unbalanced activity of lower levels that are normally under control of higher centres. It has been assumed that these inhibitory impulses originate in the motor cortex and are conducted spinalwards by cortico-spinal fibres, but there is some evidence that they depend on the release of subcortical centres owing to interruption of their cortical connections, or of injury of fibres of subcortical origin which accompany the cortico-spinal fibres in the pyramidal tracts. Whatever its exact mechanism may be the increase of tone in the muscles and exaggeration of the stretch reflexes in paretic limbs emphasises the fact that inhibition plays an essential part in the performance and co-ordination of purposive movement; it checks inappropriate reflex responses excited by stimuli from the outer world or from the limbs themselves, and associated movements unnecessary in the act are kept under control and subordinated to the will and the well-being of the body as a whole.

The functional relations of the upper and the lower motor neurons are so intimate that any acute lesion of the former depresses for a time the activity of the latter. A sudden interruption of the pyramidal tracts in the brain or spinal cord inhibits the functional activity of the spinal reflex mechanisms to such a degree that reflexes, as the knee-jerk and the tone of the muscles, may disappear for days and return only when shock has passed off. Even in the absence of structural disease functional disturbance in the cortex, as that associated with a local convulsion, may have the same effect, but in this case it is transient as the cortex recovers quickly.

THE EXTRAPYRAMIDAL SYSTEM

The Extrapyramidal System is a rather vague term applied to higher levels of the nervous system, excluding the motor area of the cortex and its projection fibres in the corticospinal tract, which are in some way concerned in the performance and regulation of motor reactions and postures more complicated than those subserved by reflexes. As generally used it includes the basal ganglia, particularly the corpus striatum and nuclei closely connected with it, such as the nucleus subthalamicus of Luys, but as the immediate projections of these are restricted to grey matter in the adjoining portion of the mid-brain, including the red nucleus, the substantia nigra and especially nuclei in the tegmentum of the mid-brain, it is not possible to consider the basal ganglia as an isolated system.

In the lowest vertebrates the corpus striatum is represented mainly by the globus pallidus or pallidum, and this has been named consequently the palæostriatum. It develops from the tween-brain, and is in these animals the highest correlation centre for motor reactions. In reptiles and birds, in which the corpus striatum attains its relatively greatest size, another element, which is represented in higher vertebrates by the putamen and caudate nucleus, is added. This is known as the neostriatum, or simply striatum. It is significant that in contrast to the pallidum it is derived from the same embryonic structure as the cortex. The two portions of the neostriatum were originally a single mass, and even in man are connected at their anterior ends, but in the greater part of their extent they are separated by fibres of the internal capsule.

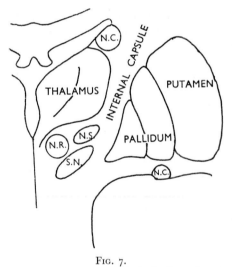

FIG. 7.

An oblique section through the brain to show the relative positions of the main extrapyramidal nuclei. N.R., red nucleus. N.S., subthalamic nucleus. S.N., substantia nigra.

A suitable section through the brain (Fig. 7) shows that all these masses of grey matter lie close together, the putamen and pallidum on the outer side of the internal capsule, the caudate nucleus and sub-thalamic nucleus between it and the thalamus. Caudal to them, and probably intimately connected with them, are the red nucleus, the substantia nigra and the nuclei and scattered cells of the tegmentum of the mid-brain.

The anatomical connections of the extrapyramidal system have not been fully worked out. All the nuclei, but particularly the striatum, receive fibres from the motor cortex and afferent impulses are also derived from the cerebellum and vestibular nuclei through the thalamus. The main route of discharge is through short neuronal links from the striatum and substantia nigra to the globus pallidus and from there to the red nucleus, subthalamic nucleus and, most importantly, to the descending reticular system in the mid-brain and medulla. The main efferent flow is through the reticulo-spinal tract but there are also important links between the globus pallidus and the ventro-lateral nucleus of the thalamus.

It is not yet possible to define the exact functions of the extrapyramidal system as a whole, or those of its separate portions. Lack of precise knowledge is due to the fact that experiments on them in animals have yielded few positive results, and observations on the effects of disease involving them in man do not justify more than vague hypotheses. Each of the separate nuclei has probably specific functions, but their exact nature is still in doubt. The functions of the red nucleus in the body righting reflexes in the cat have not been shown to be relevant to human disease. The interactions of the vestibular nuclei and the reticular formation in the brain stem in maintaining rigidity in the decerebrate cat are also not certainly applicable to man.

The functions of the substantia nigra and of the nucleus subthalamicus have not yet been ascertained, but increase of tone in all the muscles of the opposite side of the body and uncontrollable involuntary movements have resulted from disease involving them.

The corpus striatum as a whole probably integrates and co-ordinates the activities of these lower centres, and though its connections with the cerebral cortex are few, it probably participates in many of its phasic activities. The neostriatum, which is a newer structure developed from the same rudiment as the cortex, probably plays the chief part in these functions by controlling the activity of the pallidum and by integrating through it the lower centres into a smoothly working and efficient machine.

But many of the functions of the extrapyramidal system can at present be considered only in negative terms, as revealed by the disturbances which characterise disease of it in man, rather than in exact physiological terms. These disturbances, which constitute various clinical syndromes, vary with the structure involved and the nature of the lesion. Some negative symptoms, as loss of tone, slowness of voluntary movement, poverty in automatic movements and loss of associated and expressional movements, can be regarded as direct effects of destructive lesions; but positive symptoms, as the involuntary movements and increase of muscle tone which are common features of many of these diseases, must be attributed to over-activity or disordered action of unaffected parts no longer under inhibition or control, not to the effects of irritation; they often persist for years. It would, however, be absurd to include in the functions of the basal ganglia the prevention of involuntary movements.

This mixture of positive and negative symptoms is one of the difficulties encountered in attempting to reach definite conclusions on the functions of separate parts of the system. The diffuse and incomplete nature of most of the diseases that affect it, also makes difficult the correlation of disturbances of function with anatomical lesions. For instance, in Parkinsonism, which is characterised by muscular rigidity and tremor, all the basal ganglia may be involved, but the substantia nigra and the pallidum usually suffer most severely.

The state of muscle tone varies: in some conditions it is increased, in others reduced. This evidently depends on the structures which are damaged, or on the relative severity of the lesions in different parts of the system.

The increased tone differs in both distribution and character from that associated with lesions of the motor cortex and its projection fibres. It affects all muscles, and is often greatest in the trunk and neck in contrast to the spasticity of hemiplegia, which is found chiefly in the limbs, and is selective here. Further, it persists through the whole range of passive displacement, and offers to the hand that moves the limb a vibratory sensation or intermittent resistance which has been compared to that of rough cogwheels working on one another. It is not accompanied by changes in the proprioceptive and cutaneous reflexes that characterise spastic states.

Loss or diminution of tone, when it occurs, as in chorea, is also uniformly widespread. It is distinguishable from that due to section of the dorsal spinal roots, in that it often varies in intensity and that the knee-jerks and other stretch reflexes persist.

In disease of the basal ganglia and associated structures there is rarely serious reduction in the strength of movement, and even when kinetic power is diminished, static power, that is the resistance which the patient can oppose to displacement, is normal or even increased.

Voluntary movements are, however, often irregular, jerky or in-co-ordinate, and when muscle tone is increased they may be remarkably slow in both initiation and execution. This slowness may be partly due to rigidity which impedes movement, but this is not the only factor. A feature of it is that it does not extend to all movements. A man who can raise his arm only slowly and apparently with great effort may catch a ball thrown to him as quickly as a normal person, and though his gait be retarded and laboured he may jump aside promptly when in danger of being run over. Movements during sleep do not share in this slowness. I have seen a man who could scarcely walk in his waking state wander about easily in a period of somnambulism. Many patients also find they are less incapacitated for a short time after waking than during the rest of the day.

Delay in starting movements and slow performance are often particularly striking in alternating movements, as in attempting rapid pronation and supination of the forearm, polishing or rubbing, writing and beating a rhythm with the fingers. The patient is unable to switch promptly from one movement to its opposite, or even to another, especially when the attempt is prolonged, but other series of movements may be carried out more or less naturally. It may be some seconds before a man suffering with Parkinson's Disease can start to walk, but once in his stride he may continue without difficulty. He may, however, be unable to halt suddenly as a result of inabiity to adjust his centre of gravity to his base owing to rigidity of his muscles; the momentum of gait consequently carries him forward, he has to run after his centre of gravity to avoid falling.

Though in uncomplicated cases there is no paralysis of voluntary movement, reduction or absence of automatic movements, as blinking and swinging the arms in walking, is a common feature of certain extra-pyramidal syndromes. Associated movements, as flexion of the fingers of one hand when the patient grasps firmly with the other, or a tendency for one leg to extend when the other is drawn up against resistance, are also frequently absent.

Movements of expression are often affected too. A mask-like, ex-pressionless face, a statuesque attitude and diminished emotional display are common, especially in hypertonic conditions, but in other affections, as chorea, grimacing, expressional excess and restlessness occur apart from corresponding emotional states.

Many of the involuntary movements of extrapyramidal disease, as tremor, athetosis and chorea, which are dealt with in another chapter, are associated with changes in muscle tone, but the active contractions of the muscles which bring them about must be due to release or disordered activity of centres no longer under the control normally exerted on them by others. The abolition of certain involuntary movements, notably the tremor of Parkinson's disease, by circumscribed surgical lesions in the ventro-lateral nucleus of the thalamus, without any loss of motor power has not so far been satisfactorily explained but suggests that some mechanism more complex than simple release is involved. There is no conclusive evidence that any rhythmically discharging neuronal circuits are concerned in the production of Parkinsonian tremor and the concept of some higher centre having the function of suppressing such activity is not readily acceptable.

The chief indication of the functions of the extrapyramidal motor system afforded by clinical observations is that it plays an important part in the regulation and distribution of muscle tone. The motor disturbances which frequently appear when parts of it are injured suggests it is also concerned in certain motor reactions, particularly in associated and automatic movements. It also seems to facilitate and co-ordinate the co-operation of lower motor mechanisms in movements initiated at higher levels and particularly in the cerebral cortex, the precision and harmony of which are disordered by its disease. The involuntary movements that occur with many affections of the extrapyramidal system can only be attributed tentatively to disturbances in the functional equilibrium of the whole system when parts of it are injured.

Chapter V

Muscle Tone and Co-ordination of Movement

Muscle Tone

THE concept of muscular *tone* originally referred to a state of steady contraction in the unstriped muscle of hollow viscera. Its subsequent application to voluntary muscle has led to some confusion as the term has been used in several different senses. The clinician assesses the tone of the limb musculature by estimating the degree of resistance to passive movement. Provided that relaxation can be achieved, passive flexion and extension at the major joints elicits a barely detectable sense of resistance in the normal limb. This clearly cannot with confidence be attributed to any pre-existing steady "tonic" muscular contraction and, indeed, cannot by definition be detected at all unless the limb is moved. Moreover this resistance is not normally accompanied by any electrical discharge from the muscle and is certainly due in part to the physical properties of muscular tissue.

The term "postural tone" has often been applied to a state of steady muscular contraction presumed to be responsible for maintaining the upright posture. Muscular contraction is obviously involved for the paralysed patient cannot stand, but recordable activity in the anti-gravity muscles is intermittent, apparently directed to correcting deviations from the vertical and by no means resembling continuous tonic contraction.

To the physiologist the maintenance of postures clearly demanding continuous muscular contraction, such as abducting the arm, depends on the activity of *tonic* motor neurons and tonic reflexes but the term is used to contrast with the *phasic* neurons and reflexes involved in rapid movement and has little resemblance to the *tone* of the clinician.

Although these different concepts of the meaning of muscular tone are intimately linked it is clear that no simple definition is possible. If tone can conveniently be regarded as the degree of resistance to passive movement it must be remembered that this is a mere artifact of the method of examination and often but a minor sign of important disorder of function.

Apart from the small contribution of the natural elasticity of muscle, tone, as understood by the clinician, is a function of the stretch reflex. Sherrington's classical studies of the stretch reflex were necessarily and deliberately directed to the reflex arc in relative isolation from the influence of higher nervous centres. In these conditions if a muscle is stretched, even minutely, it contracts to restore its previous length. If stretch is maintained the muscle will eventually relax sufficiently to adapt to the new posture. It is easy to regard the stretch reflex and lengthening reaction as phenomena of the spinal laboratory preparation, of clinical interest only in explaining disturbances of muscle tone and tendon reflexes. The mechanisms underlying these apparently simple events are, however, to a large extent responsible for all controlled movement.

The receptor organ of the stretch reflex arc is the muscle spindle. Although further refinements are constantly being described the spindle consists essentially of a spiral sensory organ surrounding a group of small specialised motor fibres. The two ends of these intrafusal fibres can contract, while the central portion, surrounded by the sensory receptor, cannot. The sensitivity of the receptor to stretch therefore varies according to the degree of tension in the intrafusal fibres. This is largely independent of the tension in the bulk of the muscle fibres actually responsible for the contractile force of the muscle for the motor nerve supply of the two groups of fibres is quite distinct. The intrafusal supply is derived from fibres which, because of their small diameter, fall into the gamma group, but which are better referred to as fusimotor fibres. Increased firing of these fibres causes stretching of the central portion of the intrafusal muscle fibres and heightened sensitivity of the receptor organs.

Afferent impulses from the spindles pass up fast-conducting fibres some of which synapse directly or through inter-neurons with the alpha motor neurons, the anterior horn cells, and reflexly excite contraction of the muscle. If stretch is maintained impulses arise from receptor organs in the tendons which inhibit motor neuron activity and allow the muscle to lengthen.

In this grossly over-simplified account no attempt has been made to incorporate recent knowledge of the different forms of spindle receptor organs and their association with at least two distinct types of intrafusal fibre. These discoveries are of undoubted physiological importance but have not yet influenced the practice of clinical neurology.

The simplest form of stretch reflex is the monosynaptic phasic reflex, the response of the muscle to a sudden increase in tension. The functional significance of this form of response is less immediately obvious than its great importance in clinical neurology and the tendon jerks are described in detail in Chapter X. The response of the muscle to less sudden stretch, as in the clinical estimation of tone, is the result of tonic reflexes probably served by different receptor elements within the spindles and by poly-synaptic central connections.

The normal stimulus for the stretch reflex is not, of course, passive movement of the limb or a blow from a tendon hammer but the alterations in length and tension implicit in spontaneous movement. The smooth performance of any movement involves the lengthening and shortening of many muscles and the adjustment of their contraction and of the sensitivity of their spindles not only to the precise required degree but in precisely the correct sequence. Impulses arising from the spindles reflexly control muscular contraction which in turn modifies the afferent inflow. As a

D

purely spinal mechanism it is obvious that such reflex activity could neither initiate nor maintain voluntary activity. The control of the stretch reflex by higher nervous centres could theoretically be exerted either through the excitability of the alpha-motor neurons or of the fusimotor neurons and almost certainly both are important. It is even possible that the initiation of voluntary movement may not always follow the accepted pathway from cortex to anterior horn cell but that the initial event may be an alteration in the rate of fusimotor firing, leading reflexly to a change in alpha-motor neuron activity. The frequent association of disorders of muscle tone and of co-ordinated movement is readily explicable if both are dependent on the stretch reflex.

Loss of muscle tone does not in itself cause symptoms and is not always easy to detect as the stretch reflex contributes little to the perceptible resistance to passive movement of the normal limb. Hypermobility of the joints may result from loss of the normal protective reflex muscular contraction. Flaccidity inevitably results from interruption of either the afferent or efferent side of the reflex arc.

The paralysis produced by acute lesions of the central nervous system is usually initally flaccid. In both paraplegia and hemiplegia the loss of reflex activity and muscular tone is to be attributed to shock in which there is virtually complete failure of neuronal function in those parts of the nervous system isolated from their central connections. Occasionally a hemiplegia remains permanently flaccid, possibly due to a combination of lesions of the corticospinal and extrapyramidal pathways.

Destructive lesions of the cerebellum may be accompanied by hypotonicity with retention of the tendon reflexes.

Increase in muscle tone is of far greater importance because of its relative frequency, its clinical associations and the disability it causes. It takes two forms, *spasticity* and *rigidity*.

In *spasticity* the increase in resistance to passive movement is undoubtedly due to an increase in both tonic and phasic stretch reflexes. The tendon jerks are increased and rapid movement of the affected limb causes a sharp contraction of the stretched muscle followed by relaxation. In more severe degrees the resistance to passive movement may be so extreme that even by the utmost exertion it may not be possible to overcome the reflex contraction of the patient's quadriceps. Usually, however, sustained pressure results in at first gradual flexion followed by sudden relaxation—the "clasp-knife" effect. This is the lengthening reaction familiar from the spinal animal.

Spasticity due to cerebral lesions is usually maximal in the antigravity muscles, the flexors of the upper limb and extensors of the lower limb, although by no means confined to these muscles. This distribution leads to the characteristic hemiplegic gait with the toe scraping the ground and the arm held flexed against the trunk. In spinal lesions the distribution of spasticity is more variable and the degree of disability is greatly modified by the extent to which the flexors of the lower limbs are included in the heightened reflex activity. Walking is possible, although difficult, with both legs weak but spastic in extension. In many progressive lesions there is a gradual increase in reflex activity in the flexors of the hip and knee. At first the preponderance of flexor activity is intermittent and momentary, but is sufficient to cause the patient to fall. If flexor spasms increase the condition of "paraplegia-in-flexion" is eventually reached in which the lower limbs are permanently and often painfully flexed to such a degree that even sitting in a chair is impossible.

The exaggeration of spinal reflex activity is certainly due to release from the inhibition of higher centres but there is no agreement on the origin of these inhibitory impulses or on their termination. The clinical convention that interruption of the cortico-spinal pathway is the essential feature is useful but cannot be the whole answer. The reticular formation in the brain-stem undoubtedly plays an important role but as separate nuclei within this structure are known to exert opposing effects on spinal reflex activity a definitive statement would be premature. Similarly controversy still surrounds the question of whether reflex activity is increased because the alpha-motor neurons become hyperexcitable or whether the rate of fusimotor firing, and therefore the sensitivity of the spindles, is the more important factor.

Although spasticity is often taken to refer merely to the increase in tone and reflex activity the concept should certainly be widened to include the accompanying disorder of movement. A spastic limb, if not totally paralysed, is capable of a limited range of stereotyped movements, slowly and clumsily performed. The normal principle of reciprocal innervation is lacking so that, for example, an attempt to flex the limb results in powerful and inappropriate contraction of most or even all the muscles of the limb and even of the contralateral limb. To what extent this disability can be attributed to loss of function—a negative symptom—or to reflex hyper-excitability—a positive symptom—is uncertain but is of importance with regard to possible therapy.

Rigidity, the form of increased tone found in disease of the extra-pyramidal system, differs from spasticity in several respects. It is characterised by more uniform, inelastic and continuous resistance of muscles to stretching, and by an approximately equal increase of tone in all groups. Any special attitudes the limbs may assume are due to the bulk and power of the muscles rather than to unequal distribution of tone in them. Those of the trunk are affected equally, or even more severely, than those of the limbs.

Since in man it is greater when the neostriatum is damaged, or when the pallidum is less affected than it, it is probable the former controls a tonic influence of the latter and of other centres in the upper portion of the brain-stem on the muscles.

Two types of rigidity can be distinguished. In the *plastic* type the resistance to passive movement is smooth, like that experienced in bending a piece of lead. It occurs with lesions of the upper portion of the mid-brain and in catatonia. In the more common "*cogwheel rigidity*," which characterises Parkinsonism and other affections of the basal ganglia, the resistance is less uniform, it gives the impression of cogwheels moving on one another, or the sensation obtained on drawing a pencil across a corrugated surface. It is due to the intermittent yielding of muscles to stretching.

Although rigidity is certainly dependent on reflex activity, for it disappears if the dorsal spinal roots are cut, it is not accompanied by any increase in the tendon jerks—the phasic stretch reflexes. Entirely contra-dictory views on the possible role of fusimotor function have been expressed and the nature of rigidity is not understood.

CO-ORDINATION OF MOVEMENT

Co-ordination implies the execution of a movement with accuracy and the least possible expenditure of energy and of time.

Even the simplest action entails the co-operation of many muscles, and its co-ordination requires that they come into action in proper sequences and combinations, and that their contractions and relaxations are appropriately graded. Some, the agonists or prime movers, contract to execute the movement; others, the antagonists, relax or modify their tone to facilitate it; the synergics reinforce the movement and prevent displacements which may interfere with it, and the fixating muscles maintain the appropriate posture of the limb. In grasping, for instance, the hand is closed by contraction of the long and short flexors of the fingers, but their extensors relax reciprocally; the extensors of the wrist contract to prevent the wrist flexing and thus enfeebling the grasp, and the limb is held in the proper position by tonic contraction of muscles acting on the elbow and shoulder joints. Failure of any of these factors disturbs the accuracy of the action.

The precision and accurate adaptation of movements and motor reactions may be interfered with by various abnormalities of motor and other functions of the nervous system. Weakness of a limb of any nature may impair the accuracy of its movements; those of a spastic limb are jerky and defectively proportioned; involuntary movements may deviate it from its natural course; defective postural fixation of parts on which the limb moves leads to deviations from the direct line, and in the absence of sensory guidance by impulses of proprioceptive origin both the direction and range of movement may be defective.

When owing to injury or disease of the nervous system an action cannot be carried out in an ordinary or natural manner attempts to attain its end by other means may also result in clumsy and irregular movements.

In clinical practice, however, the terms inco-ordination or ataxia are restricted to conditions in which lack of accuracy and proper grading are not due to paresis, spasticity or involuntary movements, or to round-about modes of performance.

Co-ordination does not depend on any one centre or part, it is a function of the nervous system as a whole. Even the simplest reflexes obtainable in the spinal animal are co-ordinated; the scratch reflex of the spinal dog is an example of the appropriateness and accuracy of response to a peripheral stimulus.

The more complicated activities of the intact animal demand more elaborate mechanisms. This is provided in the upper part of the hind-brain and possibly in the basal ganglia, too, one of the functions of which is the regulation of posture and equilibrium during rest and in motion by muscular contractions and modifications of muscle tone.

Motor responses to stimulation of the cerebral cortex are also co-ordinate, and so are those initiated here either reflexly or by volition. This depends partly on subcortical centres which co-operate with the cortex in movement, but in the cortex itself the elementary or fractional movements represented in its motor area are properly graded and combined into purposive acts. Cortical co-ordination depends largely on impulses which supply information on the initial posture and on the range and direction of the movement during its successive phases. The movements of a limb in which postural sensation is defective are ill-directed and ill-adapted to their aim. These irregularities, which are generally included in the term *sensory ataxia*, can be to some extent controlled by other senses, and especially by vision; they are greater when vision is excluded in contrast to the inco-ordination which results from lesions of lower levels on which vision has no influence.

The importance of afferent impulses that do not reach consciousness, particularly from the muscle spindles, has already been emphasised. The cerebellum appears to be the most important centre where such impulses are integrated with those derived from all the other afferent systems of the body and from the motor and sensory cortex. The efferent flow, carrying the results of this integration, is widely relayed to the thalamus, the extrapyramidal system, the cerebral cortex and the spinal cord. The symptoms and signs of cerebellar disease can be largely attributed to failure of the normal integration between the fusimotor system and effective muscular contraction. The precisely graded and timed contraction and relaxation of many muscles implicit in any voluntary movement are no longer possible.

The irregularities of movement of cerebellar disease can be most easily studied when they are due to an acute unilateral lesion. Muscle tone is diminished, as shown by the flaccidity and abnormal extensibility of the muscles on the same side of the body, and particularly loss of postural fixation owing to which a limb fails to maintain steadily its position when unsupported and to adapt its posture to changing conditions during movement (Fig. 8). Failure of immobilisation and of appropriate variations in the contraction of the muscles of the proximal segments of a limb is one of the causes of deviations from the direct line of movement which is a feature of cerebellar ataxia.

In acute stages voluntary movements are enfeebled, but to a slight degree only. As stimulation of the cerebellum lowers the threshold of excitability of the opposite motor cortex, it seems that it in some way augments the cortical motor apparatus. Paresis is, however, rarely a prominent symptom even in acute disease, and never persists for long. There may also be a short delay in both starting and arresting movements, and spontaneous movements are often slower and more deliberate than those of a normal limb.

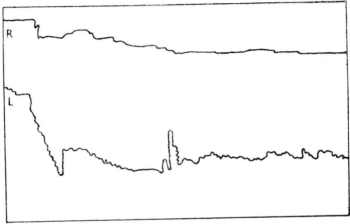

FIG. 8.

A support was suddenly withdrawn from the two outstretched arms of a man in whom there was an acute lesion of the left side of the cerebellum. The left arm fell at once through a larger angle and developed irregular tremor.

Owing to deficiency of the normal correcting mechanisms unsupported parts of the body, as the head and outstretched limbs, are commonly tremulous, for voluntary effort alone fails to preserve steady posture (Fig. 8). Voluntary movements are often jerky or irregular in rate, apparently owing to incomplete fusion of the impulses that produce tetanic contractions of the muscles (Fig. 9).

Further, the range of purposive movements is frequently inaccurate; the hand overshoots the point it wishes to reach, owing to either delay in arresting the movement, or to lack of co-ordinated contraction in the antagonists which normally steady and control it. The importance of the latter factor is shown by the fact that if the hand is thrown passively towards the face it may strike it forcibly, even when the patient, as a result of previous experiences, tries to arrest the limb. Absence or delayed intervention of the antagonists is also seen in the "rebound phenomenon";

when a normal forearm is flexed against resistance the excursion of the limb is quickly checked when the resistance is suddenly released, but the affected arm moves till arrested by the ligaments or by opposition of the surfaces of the joint.

Frequently, however, the hand or foot stops short of the point the patient wishes to reach, and then approaches it by a series of irregular jerks. Failure to bring the hand directly to its object may sometimes be due to voluntary arrest when a patient has learned that he is liable to pass beyond it, but it is more often a primary result of defective grading of movement.

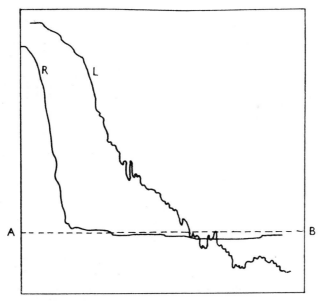

Fig. 9.

Tracings obtained on a moving drum of the attempts of a patient with a lesion of the left side of the cerebellum to touch a point represented by the line A—B. Movement of the left arm was slower, more irregular and tremulous, and the finger was not arrested when it reached the point.

These disturbances are particularly obvious in the performance of alternating movements, as rapid pronation and supination of the forearm; the individual excursions are irregular in rate and range, there is delay in switching from one movement to the next, and unless the elbow is held firmly to the side or rests on a support, the limb sways about irregularly (Fig. 10).

Owing to these primary disturbances voluntary movements lack their normal smoothness, and are irregular in direction, rate and range. Unlike the errors due to loss of sensation they cannot be corrected by visual guidance, and are equally pronounced whether the patient's eyes are open or closed.

Associated movements are usually affected too; while walking the arm of the affected side does not swing, and vigorous contraction of the muscles of a normal limb may not be accompanied by innervation of those of the affected side.

Injury of the cerebellum affects all voluntary movements. Nystagmus on deviation of the eyes is due to failure to maintain them in the position to which they are moved; articulation and phonation become slow, irregular and jerky, and, as may be seen when the patient attempts to sing, even voluntary movements of the chest may be disordered, but this is more obvious when both sides of the cerebellum are involved.

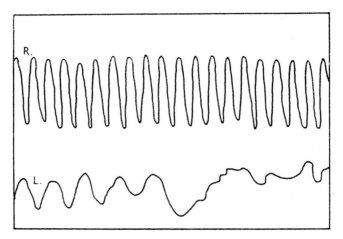

FIG. 10.

Tracings of alternating pronation and supination of the right (R) and left (L) forearms in a case of injury of the left side of the cerebellum. At first the movements of the left forearm were only slower and smaller in range, but became irregular and ceased with the arm in supination.

The characteristic symptoms of cerebellar disease also appear when its connections in the pons and mid-brain are injured, but then they are usually accompanied by other disturbances.

Experiments on animals indicate there may be separate representation of different portions of the body on the surface of the cerebellum comparable to that in the cortex of the forebrain, but clinical experience provides little evidence of it. The disorders of movement that result from injury of one side are limited to the limbs of the same side, but bilateral symptoms, particularly defective co-ordination of movements of the trunk which are necessary for maintenance of the erect posture of the body in walking, are prominent in affections of its middle lobe or vermis. This is because the afferent fibres from the vestibular system, concerned with the maintenance of balance, are projected to this region. In extreme cases the patient can neither walk, stand or even sit upright and yet the function of the limbs when tested individually appears normal. This is a fruitful source for the erroneous diagnosis of hysteria.

The symptoms of acute cerebellar disease tend to subside gradually; the execution of delicate and complicated actions, and those requiring change in rate and direction of movement, are, as a rule, the last to recover.

Two or more factors may combine to disturb the co-ordination of movement. The ataxia of tabes dorsalis, for instance, may be due to hypotonia of the muscles owing to interruption of spinal reflex arcs, to loss of postural sensation, or to absence of afferent impulses to higher levels as those conveyed to the cerebellum by the cells of Clarke's column and the spinocerebellar tracts. These factors vary from patient to patient. In many cases loss of sensation explains it adequately, but in others the ataxia is so great in relation to the sensory disturbance that it must be attributed to interruption of other afferent impulses to supraspinal levels.

Chapter VI

Involuntary Movements

INVOLUNTARY and uncontrollable movements are a common symptom of nervous disease. Some are associated with structural lesions of the brain and others with systemic metabolic disorders, but in all but the simplest forms the underlying disturbance of physiology is obscure. Most of them can be interpreted as manifestations of disorder in the functional equilibrium of parts concerned in the regulation of muscle tone or in the execution of certain categories of movement.

If those of psychological origin be excluded all possess the features that they are useless, purposeless and in no way adapted to the patient's needs, and that they cannot be arrested, or at the most checked for a short time only, by his efforts. Different types are distinguished by their characters and by the factors that determine their onset or modify them. Most cease during sleep and in complete muscular relaxation; in some the tone of the muscles is increased, in others diminished; some persist in voluntary movement and disorder it, others disappear during active use of the limb and most are aggravated by emotional disturbances. Though the affected limbs may be weak, all except those of reflex nature disappear with the onset of loss of voluntary power.

The only common involuntary movements due to affection of peripheral motor nerves result from faulty reinnervation of the facial muscles after a facial palsy. If the nerve has degenerated the axons must grow again and some inevitably terminate on muscle fibres other than those they originally supplied and may even enter different muscles. With most nerves this is of no importance but the facial nerve supplies many small muscles whose function of minutely controlling the facial expression ensures that the effects of faulty innervation are obvious. Voluntary closure of the eye may be weak and yet full closure may occur involuntarily every time the patient smiles. Associated movements of this kind may sometimes be so extensive that the entire facial musculature may contract simultaneously, and inappropriately on any attempted movement.

This form of facial spasm, that follows any severe peripheral facial palsy, must be distinguished from the many forms of involuntary movement of the facial muscles of central origin and also from clonic facial spasm. This is not a sequel of facial palsy but may result from irritative lesions of the facial nerve within the skull. The muscles of one side of the face, particularly those around the eye, contract frequently and irregularly, not as a disorganisation of voluntary movement, but spontaneously and involuntarily.

Reflex spasmodic contractions of muscles also result from irritating lesions of sensory nerves. Any sudden pain, as those of tabes dorsalis, may excite abrupt involuntary movements. Spasm of the face is so striking a feature of severe bouts of trigeminal neuralgia that this has become known as "tic douloureux."

It is doubtful if long continuing involuntary movements are ever directly due to irritative lesions of the central nervous system, as tumours, scars or inflammatory foci. Those which occur with central disease fall into two classes. The first includes reflexes, either normal but exaggerated, or pathological in the sense that they are not seen under natural conditions. The cramps and spasms of spastic limbs are essentially reflex. They are excited by cutaneous or proprioceptive impulses acting on spinal centres which are over-active owing to not being under the control of higher levels. The clonus which often develops in spastic limbs is due to stretch or tension on hypertonic muscles by external forces or by gravity.

The second class includes movements which are usually more complex and unlike normal motor reactions. They are not excited or materially influenced by peripheral stimuli. As they are positive symptoms, or products of over-activity, they cannot be directly due to the destructive or degenerative lesions with which they are associated. It is generally accepted that the impulses which produce them arise from the over-activity of parts of the central motor apparatus which, owing to disease, are released or freed from the control or inhibition normally exerted on them by the damaged structures. This hypothesis of release explains many of these abnormal and apparently spontaneous movements, but release should lead to the appearance, though in exaggerated form, of activities in some way related to the ordinary function of the part, as the flexor spasms that withdraw a spastic limb from a stimulus. Some are, however, wholly unlike anything seen in natural conditions, and are lacking in any trace of purpose or aim. They can most easily be explained by disorganisation of the complicated extrapyramidal and postural systems in which the chief pathological changes are found. In most cases these changes are diffuse, and involve more or less the same structures regardless of the nature of the movements. The form the latter assume is probably determined by the relative severity of the affection of different parts. When the main stress of the disease falls on one part disturbing one functional component and releasing others we have chorea, when on other parts athetosis, torsion spasm or tremor.

The corticospinal system seems to be of secondary importance in the pathogenesis of these types of involuntary movement, provided it is not so gravely injured as to produce a severe degree of paralysis.

Many of these involuntary movements are associated with striking changes in the tone of the muscles of the affected parts. The writhings and contortions of athetosis result from series of tonic contractions of varying groups of muscles; static tremor is often accompanied by persisting rigidity, as in the Parkinsonian syndrome, and chorea by hypotonicity of muscles.

The more common forms of involuntary movements are those generally known as chorea, athetosis and tremor, but these types may be intermixed, and not infrequently it is difficult to decide to which category they belong.

Choreic movements are forcible rapid jerks of short duration and variable distribution which never combine into a co-ordinate act. They may involve all parts of the body, or be limited to one side, to a limb, to one side of the face or to the bulbar musculature. All reactive and expressive movements of the affected parts are exaggerated, and voluntary movements are usually excessive and irregular, partly as they are disturbed by spasms, partly owing to defective fixation of the limbs which are almost invariably hypotonic. They appear in their most typical form in Sydenham's chorea, but they also occur in Huntington's disease, with inflammatory lesions of the basal ganglia as epidemic encephalitis, with local softenings, and in degenerative conditions as hepato-lenticular degeneration. These are the only involuntary movements that commonly occur in sleep.

Athetosis is characterised by slow, sinuous and purposeless movements which often start in the distal segments of a limb and spread to the proximal, but they may involve the trunk, face and neck. They are frequently unilateral. The individual movements are of longer duration than those of chorea, and often become confluent leading to grotesque postures which may not be possible by willed effort. Athetotic movements are intermittent. During the spasms all the muscles of the affected part are in strong tonic contraction, and produce typical postures, as separation and over-extension of the fingers, which change slowly in mobile spasm.

Reactionary movements are easily excited and tend to have the same excessive, grotesque character. Willed movements of the affected limbs or strong innervation of another limb may bring on spasms.

Torsion spasm is allied to athetosis; it may succeed it or both may be present at the same time. Its special feature is exceptionally strong tonic contractions of muscles of the trunk, neck and of the proximal segments of the limbs, which produce a variety of contortions, as retraction of the head, excessive lordosis, rotation of the trunk and weird movements of whole limbs. At rest there may be a few or no spasms, but they appear on voluntary movement. In the spasms the limbs become rigid, but they are usually flaccid at rest.

In the rare condition known as *hemiballismus*, the involuntary movements, which are limited to one side, are even larger, wilder and more forcible. The proximal segments of the limbs and trunk are chiefly involved. Its main interest is that it is one of the few forms which result from small focal lesions; the nucleus subthalamicus is almost always damaged, usually by a softening.

By far the commonest form of involuntary movement is *tremor*, consisting of more or less regular, rhythmic contractions of muscles and their antagonists. Many different types may be distinguished by their frequency and distribution and by their relationship with voluntary movement. As a rule tremor is most pronounced in the distal segments of the limbs but may involve the head, trunk, face and even the bulbar muscles. The tremor of Parkinson's disease is characteristically at a rate around 4 to 6 per second and persists even when the limb is fully supported. It may be less obvious during voluntary action but is usually increased by strong movements of the other limbs. Like all forms of tremor it is exaggerated by emotional tension and also fluctuates greatly in degree for no apparent cause. In contrast, hereditary essential tremor is absent at rest and is most pronounced when the patient attempts to maintain a fixed posture.

Of great interest are those forms of tremor due to reversible metabolic disorders rather than to destructive cerebral lesions. The rapid tremor of thyrotoxicosis and the more violent movements of delirium tremens have long been known. More recently a characteristic flapping tremor of the outstretched hands has been observed in liver disease. An irregular and infrequent tremor of the hands is sometimes seen in carbon dioxide retention in chronic lung disease.

Reversible Parkinsonian rigidity and tremor are readily produced by chronic treatment with phenothiazine drugs and more rarely unusual forms of involuntary movement may occur as the acute effects of overdosage. Torsion spasm, trismus and forced deviation of the eyes (oculogyric crises) and many other forms have been observed and the relationship between metabolism and structural lesions in the causation of involuntary movements is emphasised by the occasional development of persistent intractable movements as the result of phenothiazine therapy.

Palatal myoclonus consists of regular rhythmic elevation of the soft palate, sometimes accompanied by synchronous contractions of the pharyngeal muscles and vocal cords. The return of the palate to its position of rest is due to gravity, not to contraction of the antagonists of the elevators.

Myoclonus is characterised by sudden abrupt, often isolated contractions of a muscle, of part of a muscle or of several muscles regardless of their functional association; they occur irregularly in time and distribution, but the muscles of the limbs are involved more frequently than those of the trunk and head. The twitches resemble those which are excited by an electrical stimulus; frequently they produce no movement.

Although this description may appear sufficiently distinctive the term has been applied with little discrimination to a great variety of shock-like involuntary movements of differing aetiology. A broad distinction is possible between the epileptic and non-epileptic forms, although even these may occur in the same patient. To avoid confusion it is often better to describe what is seen rather than hope that the use of a stereotyped term will always convey a precise meaning.

Spasmodic Torticollis, characterised by intermittent vigorous contractions of the muscles that turn the head to one side, has been regarded as a psychopathic condition, but its occurence with symptoms of undoubtedly organic nature and as a sequel of encephalitis indicate it is a form of dystonia due to disturbances in the extrapyramidal motor system though no anatomical changes have been constantly found in it.

Tics and Habit Spasms are sudden, brief, recurrent, inappropriate and often irresistible movements which may be either simple or consist of complexes of movements in which purpose or aim is often apparent. They are, as their English name signifies, of psychological origin; the original movements, which may have been voluntary or automatic, become stereotyped, but in time are frequently modified or caricatured. Their psychological basis is their most important feature; the movements are compulsive, and can be checked for a short time only by effort of will, but an attempt to do so produces a feeling of tension which soon becomes intolerable, but is relieved by repetition of the movement.

Tics usually become more pronounced during emotional upsets, and lessen when the patient is not under observation, or when his attention is diverted from them; the latter is an important point in their distinction from choreic movements with which they may be confused.

While there can be no doubt that most types of involuntary movement result from disease or dysfunction of the subcortical masses of grey matter which are generally included in the extrapyramidal motor system, it is rarely possible owing to the diffuse and extensive pathological changes that are found to determine the essential causal lesion, or to correlate the symptoms with disease of any structure. With the exception of hemiballismus, which is almost invariably associated with softening of the nucleus subthalamicus, and of palatal myoclonus, in which only degeneration of the central tegmental tract and inferior olive are usually present, few of them are associated with focal disease.

The collation of numerous clinical and pathological observations provides, however, some evidence of the structures disease of which may result in the appearance of different varieties.

Rhythmic tremor may follow damage of the cerebello-thalamic connections, particularly when the red nucleus and the infrathalamic region are involved. Degeneration of the cells of the substantia nigra and pallidum seem to be the most important and constant change in paralysis agitans.

Scattered lesions in the basal ganglia, and often in the cortex too, have been found associated with choreiform movements. In Huntington's disease, in which they appear in characteristic form, the chief change is degeneration of the small cells of the striatum.

In acquired unilateral athetosis lesions have been found in the cerebello-thalamic system; in the congenital or infantile disease changes occur in both the striatum and cortex. Disease of the striatum, nucleus subthalamicus and red nucleus has been described in torsion spasm.

Degenerative lesions have been observed in the cerebellum, inferior olives, mid-brain nuclei and striatum in cases of myoclonus.

The remarkable effects of surgery in abolishing certain forms of involuntary movement have proved difficult to interpret. It is sometimes tempting to consider whether almost any form of interruption of the afferent flow to the extrapyramidal system might not prove effective in the abolition of tremor. It is evident that our knowledge of the lesions essential for the appearance of most forms of involuntary movement is imperfect; and of their pathological physiology we know even less, and can hope to understand their nature more fully only when the functions of the individual masses of grey matter in the basal ganglia and mid-brain, and the significance of their combined activities in the economy of posture and movement, have been unravelled.

Chapter VII

Examination of the Motor System

THE most rational method to follow in examination of the motor system is to investigate in the following order: (i) The size of the muscles, as it is largely on this that the power of motion depends; (ii) the tone of the muscles, as if this is disordered it may affect not only the execution and accuracy of movement, but also influence the exertion of power; (iii) the strength of contraction of separate muscles and groups of muscles, and of the movements they produce; (iv) the co-ordination of movement; and (v) finally, the presence or absence of involuntary or so-called spontaneous movements.

Size and Development of Muscles

The development of the musculature varies greatly in different individuals, and as such is of little significance in the investigation of disease. It depends on natural endowment, on the mode of life and on training or occupation.

Atrophy, or diminution in size, of a muscle or group of muscles in comparison with the rest of the musculature is usually pathological. It is commonly due to disintegration and disappearance of the muscle fibres, either from primary disease of the muscle or secondary to lesions of the lower motor neuron. Disuse from any cause such as immobilisation of a limb, joint disease or a severed tendon causes atrophy due to a diffuse reduction in fibre diameter.

As the bulk of an atrophied muscle depends on the reaction of its connective tissue as well as on the proportion of its contractile fibres which remain, it is important to compare its power of contraction with its apparent size. In some forms of muscular dystrophy the calf muscles, in particular, may be larger than normal, although obviously weak. This *pseudohypertrophy* is due to infiltration of the muscle with fat and also to the presence of many abnormal giant muscle fibres. In the atrophy of disuse and that around diseased joints, on the other hand, the power of contraction is often surprisingly good in relation to the size of the muscles.

Valuable information may often be obtained by palpation. Normal muscle, unless covered by a thick layer of fat, feels semi-elastic, and regains its shape at once when compressed or displaced, and fingers drawn firmly across it may receive the impression of passing over a fascicular or corrugated substance. Degenerated muscle feels softer, less elastic and more uniform in structure. When there is an overgrowth of the fibrous stroma the muscle is hard and inelastic, it cannot be displaced readily, and it is not possible to stretch it to the normal extent by movement of the joint on which it acts.

The distribution of atrophy may indicate its cause. Wasting may be restricted to the distribution of a single motor nerve or anterior root. When it is secondary to disease of a joint only those around the joint are involved, as the deltoid in case of arthritis of the shoulder and of the quadriceps extensor when the knee is diseased.

The methods of examining the nature and degree of muscular weakness by comparing the effects of Galvanic and Faradic stimulation have been replaced by the more precise techniques of the strength/duration curve, electromyography and motor nerve conduction tests. Although their description lies beyond the scope of this book the purpose of these investigations should be understood. With their aid it is possible to obtain a reliable distinction between conduction block, with an absolutely good prognosis, and denervation, with inevitably delayed and often imperfect recovery. It is possible to determine whether the degree of denervation is increasing or whether recovery has begun. Electromyography will often distinguish between primary muscle disease and the effects of a lower motor neuron lesion. Motor nerve conduction tests may indicate diffuse disease of the peripheral nervous system or localised nerve compression.

The state of reflexes in which under normal conditions the atrophied muscles are concerned is a critical distinction on the nature of the wasting. When all, or a large proportion of, the fibres are degenerated their reflex contractions excited by superficial stimuli and those evoked by a sudden stretch disappear or are abnormally depressed. In the wasting of disuse and in that which occurs around diseased joints, on the other hand, the reflexes, and especially the stretch reflexes, persist and are often exaggerated.

Fibrillation is the spontaneous contraction of individual fibres that occurs in denervated muscle in response to circulating acetylcholine and is not a clinical sign, being only detectable with the electromyograph. *Fasciculation* consists of spontaneous contraction of individual motor units. This frequently occurs in normal people, especially in the muscles of the calves, and is of no significance except that it may occasion alarm in those aware of the more sinister possibilities. Fasciculation is a classical and almost constant sign of motor neuron disease in which the surviving motor units may be greatly enlarged by the innervation of muscle fibres previously supplied by degenerated neurons. These giant units discharge spontaneously in a chaotic manner producing an irregular flickering contraction in the affected muscles. This is only rarely sufficiently strong to cause movement of the limb. It can usually be increased by percussion of the muscle or by active or passive movement. Fasciculation of this type occurs less constantly in other forms of chronic partial loss of anterior horn cells and also in peripheral lesions of the motor units, notably chronic peripheral neuropathy.

E

MUSCLE TONE

The different concepts of muscle tone were discussed in Chapter V. It was concluded that the state of steady contraction originally implied seldom occurred in voluntary muscle and a more dynamic interpretation of muscle tone was advanced. The clinician can attempt to estimate the degree of resistance to passive movement of the limbs and can also detect any accompanying disorders of the reflex control of co-ordinated muscular action.

Flaccidity, or loss or diminution of tone, may result from lesions of the spinal reflex arc, from depression of reflex activity by shock, from disorders of certain higher centres as the cerebellum, and in states of unconsciousness.

It is recognised clinically by lack of resistance to passive movement, often accompanied by excessive mobility of the part. Toneless muscles also feel soft and flabby when palpated, but this feature is too indefinite and unreliable for clinical purposes.

The first essential is to make the patient relax the part under examination, for voluntary contraction of muscles may obscure lack of their tone. The limb should then be moved about in all directions by the examiner, who during the movements estimates the resistance he meets; in a flaccid limb the only resistance in excursions of normal range is that due to its weight.

The following tests also reveal deficiency of reflex control of muscular contraction. If of mild degree it is more easily recognised when the flaccid is compared with a normal limb.

When the limb is unsupported it fails to keep its position with natural steadiness (Fig. 8); this becomes more obvious if the patient, or the chair in which he sits, is shaken abruptly.

The extended limbs, which should be fully relaxed, are placed by the patient horizontally in front of him with his hands or feet resting on the observer's hands or on a bar. On suddenly removing the support a normal limb sags a little but quickly regains its position, a flaccid limb falls through a wider angle and usually fails to come back so accurately (Fig. 8).

When the unsupported limb is tapped it sways more widely than a normal limb. In this, as in other tests, it is essential that it is not firmly braced by voluntary effort; when, for instance, the arm is examined the elbow should not be rigidly extended and muscular effort should be the minimum necessary to keep it in position. Swaying is greater when the limb is displaced in the horizontal plane, as a tap in the vertical plane encounters the resistance of the voluntary muscular contractions by which it is held up. In these two tests it is advisable that the patient closes his eyes, as if he anticipates removal of support or a tap he may brace his limbs.

If a flaccid limb, held by either a proximal or distal segment, is shaken to and fro the passive swing of its unsupported segments is greater than normal.

Hypotonic limbs often occupy unnatural attitudes, or at least attitudes which would be uncomfortable in a normal limb.

The state of the tendon jerks distinguishes the hypotonicity of cerebellar and brain-stem lesions from those due to disturbances of the spinal reflex arc, as in the latter they are lost.

Increase of muscle tone, or hypertonicity, is more easily recognised, but there is a risk that voluntary contraction may be mistaken for it. Steps must be taken to assure relaxation. This may be done by requesting the patient to allow his limbs to lie or hang beside him as if he were going to sleep, or by diverting his attention. Experience soon enables the clinician to recognise voluntary contractions.

A distinguishing feature of hypertonicity of every nature is the maintenance of postures, usually in unnatural attitudes, which are determined partly by the distribution of tone, partly by the bulk and power of the affected muscles. The critical feature, however, is excessive resistance to passive movement or displacement.

In the *spastic limb* this is usually greater in the initial stage of movement, and often diminishes or disappears when it is continued, sometimes, in fact, the muscle relaxes suddenly and its antagonists contract; this often occurs on flexing a spastic knee. The resistance is usually greater on displacement in some directions than in others, according to the distribution of tone in the muscles. The degree of spasticity varies greatly, being increased by cold, excitement or discomfort and by prolonged immobility of the limbs as in sitting.

Rigidity of both the plastic and cogwheel types offers an unvarying resistance to passive displacement, which is approximately equal in movements in all directions and throughout their whole range. It is not materially modified by external stimuli. The limbs also tend to remain in positions in which they are placed. In plastic rigidity the resistance is smooth and uniform; in the "cogwheel type" it is irregular and gives to the observer's hand a sensation of vibration.

Owing to fibrosis hypertonic muscles frequently undergo contracture or shortening which impedes stretching; this is recognised by restriction of the range of movement and by the abrupt, unyielding resistance encountered on manipulation by the examiner. In extreme examples only a general anaesthetic will permit distinction between contracture and severe spasticity.

Active Movement

When the size of the muscles and the state of their tone have been observed active movement can be investigated. This requires observation of (i) the range, and (ii) the power of movement, (iii) its rate and regularity, and (iv) the execution of complex or compound in addition to simple movements.

The range of movement may be limited by changes in joints and by fibrosis or contractures in muscles. Excessive tone in muscles may also restrict it. Weakness, too, is often accompanied by limitation of range of voluntary movement.

Power of movement.—Lesions of the central nervous system disturb movements in which several muscles are generally engaged, and it consequently suffices to test the strength of movements, as flexion or extension of the fingers or of the forearm, by observing the force necessary to restrain them against the patient's maximal effort. This naturally varies greatly in different individuals, so pathological weakness is detected more easily by comparing the same movement on the two sides if one only is involved, or by contrasting it with other movements. Dynamometers, or instruments for measuring the power exerted, are necessary only to indicate variations in voluntary power during progress of disease or recovery.

A distinction should be made between kinetic power, that is, the force. exerted in changing position, and static power or that which resists change of posture. When, for instance, an arm is raised to the horizontal it exerts kinetic power; when it resists depression or holds up a weight it does static work. In most forms of disease kinetic and static power are equally affected, and either can be tested to determine the power exerted by muscles, but in certain conditions, particularly in those due to lesions of the basal ganglia, as Parkinsonism, the former may be reduced though the latter is normal or almost so.

Muscles weak from any cause tire quickly. This fatigue is, however, different from that of *myasthenia gravis* where a muscle made to contract at frequent intervals becomes rapidly but temporarily paralysed.

In *myotonic* muscular dystrophy the remarkable phenomenon of myotonia may be seen in delayed muscular relaxation, most commonly in the hand grip. On repeated contraction myotonia disappears and muscular relaxation becomes temporarily normal.

When lower motor neurons are affected it is necessary to test the power of individual muscles, as in many instances only some of those taking part in a movement are involved. This can be done by palpating each muscle, or by feeling if its tendon tightens, when movements in which it contracts under normal conditions are attempted. The clearest indication of paresis of a muscle, however, is loss or feebleness of that component of a movement for which it is responsible, but it must not be forgotten that when a muscle is paralysed the patient may learn to employ another instead of it. The investigation of muscular palsies therefore requires knowledge of the action of each muscle.

Rate and Regularity of Movement.—The rate and regularity of voluntary and spontaneous movements are frequently disturbed by disease of the central nervous system. Limbs which are weak usually move more slowly than normal, partly due to delay in the start of movement, partly to its retarded rate. But this occurs in other conditions too: in Parkinsonism, for instance, both the initiation and execution of movements are slow, but unless the disease is severe the patient can speed it up on making a deliberate effort.

Irregularities in rate, due to ataxia or to tremor during movement have been dealt with in another section (p. 40). Feeble limbs, and particularly those in which muscle tone is excessive, often fail to move with the uniformity which characterises normal parts owing to either irregularities in the contractions of the prime movers or to intermittent relaxations of their antagonists. In rigidity associated with disease of parts of the extrapyramidal system movements are often jerky and irregular, though power may not be reduced.

A special type of irregular muscular contraction is frequently found in hysterical and other psychogenic conditions. The exertion of power is intermittent; on reaching a certain degree it suddenly relaxes, then the patient makes further spasmodic efforts, and if urged repeatedly may exert almost normal power. Another common feature of psychogenic paresis is failure to complete the movement desired, whether it is opposed or not. If asked to touch an object with a paretic limb, the finger or toe is often arrested before reaching it, then falls away and succeeds only after repeated attempts. The movements of the hysterical patient also give the impression of lacking the honest and sustained endeavour which characterises those of a pathologically weak limb.

Co-ordination of movement can be observed in the patient's ordinary activities and in specially selected tests. The latter should, in the first instance, be so simple as to make possible an analysis of the features they may present.

The two chief causes of ataxia or inco-ordination are defects in postural sensation, and disturbances in the complex co-ordinating mechanisms of the hind-brain and cerebellum. The latter are controlled by afferent impulses which do not excite sensation. When inco-ordination is present the first task, therefore, is to find out it if is accompanied by disturbances of sensation, and especially by disturbances of postural sensibility, for if a person is unaware of the point from which his limb starts and of its positions in space during successive stages of movement, naturally he cannot bring it accurately to an object he wishes to touch, but this failure to do so is not necessarily due to inco-ordination. As vision may provide the necessary information movements within its range are more accurate. In testing co-ordination, therefore, the eyes should not at first be closed or bandaged, but it is advisable to repeat the tests with vision excluded.

The usual test applied to the upper limb is to ask the patient to touch a point, or to move his finger from one point to another, deliberately and at a moderate rate. As defective vision, diplopia, or a squint with erroneous projection may misrepresent the position in space of the target, it is advisable that one of the points to be touched should be his nose or a part of his own body. A useful test is to bring his forefinger from the observer's finger to his own nose, and then reverse the movement, or touch a point with his toe and then bring his heel to the opposite knee. Finer and more delicate movements can be tested by asking the patient to bring the tip of each finger in succession to the top of his thumb, and by observing how he uses tools, as a pen or scissors, or handles objects.

The analysis of ataxia is difficult by ordinary clinical methods, but attention should be directed to its chief features. Deviations from the correct line of movement often result from defective postural fixation of proximal segments of the limb which permits it to sway about, and from a tendency to divide up a compound movement involving displacements at two or more joints into simpler components. This occurs in cerebellar disease. Errors in the range of movement, either a tendency to pass the point aimed at, or to arrest the limb before reaching it, which also occurs with cerebellar disturbance and in spastic limbs, indicate a failure to grade the muscular contractions or to check them appropriately. They are usually more prominent in rapidly executed than in slow movements.

Tremor during movement may be a manifestation of ataxia, or due to persistence of a tremor which occurs at rest. Normal movements start gradually, quickly attain a more or less uniform rate and terminate rapidly on approaching their end. During the greater part of their range tremor may cause little disability, but if it occurs towards the end of movement it interferes with its accuracy. This may be due to persistence of tremor that occurs at rest, but if the result of failure of the rate of movement to decrease at a uniform rate it is evidence of inco-ordination. Terminal tremor, often known as "intention tremor", occurs with various lesions of the central nervous system, particularly with those involving the cerebellum and brain-stem.

Ataxia is often more obvious in rapidly alternating than in individual movements; the transition from one movement to its opposite may be delayed, the range of the excursions irregular, their natural rhythm lost and prolonged attempts often lead to confusion and cessation (Fig. 10). It can be observed in various tests as pronation and supination of the forearm, flexion and extension of the fingers, or of the knee and ankle. Though each movement may be of normal range and power the patient may be unable to alternate them with normal rhythm or rapidity. This disability is a well-known feature of cerebellar disease, but it occurs also with disorders of the extra-pyramidal system, particularly in the Parkinsonian syndrome. Disturbances of tone and spasticity of even moderate degree also interfere with the rate and rhythm of alternating movements.

All motor functions may become inco-ordinate as a result of disease. Articulation, swallowing and respiration may be affected in the same manner as the limbs. Careful observation, and especially existence of disturbance of function without paresis, usually indicate the nature of the disorder.

CHAPTER VIII

Sensation

IN any description of the sensory aspects of the nervous system it is impossible to avoid writing of pathways concerned with specific sensations. It must not be forgotten, however, that no sensation exists until it is perceived and that it is nerve impulses no different from others that are transmitted and not sensations.

Under normal conditions every sensation depends on impulses excited by adequate stimulation of receptors or end-organs and conveyed to the central nervous system by afferent or sensory fibres.

All sensory structures contain such receptors. Those in the skin respond to external agents or to change in environment which affect the surface of the body, and they are consequently known as exteroceptors; those in deeper tissues which react to changes within the body are called proprioceptors. Some receptors are merely freely branching naked filaments of nerve fibres, others are highly organised structures.

In the skin terminal fine unmyelinated ramifications of fibres form a network or plexus beneath the epidermis, but some penetrate between cells of the epidermis and may even enter its cells. Much more complex receptors are present, including the basket-like nerve endings around hair follicles, Merkel's cells and Meissner's corpuscles and the end bulbs of Krause and Ruffini. Many of these appear to be structurally adapted to respond to specific stimuli and yet there is no conclusive proof that the network of unspecialised fibres respond to pain and the discrete receptors to touch, pressure and thermal stimuli.

The proprioceptive receptors, on which knowledge of what is happening within our bodies depends, include muscle-spindles and Golgi tendon organs which are excited by tension and stretch in muscles, and Pacinian corpuscles in subcutaneous tissues, joints and visceral organs, which probably respond to pressure.

Anatomical methods have shown that a single nerve fibre may supply several end-organs; branches of one fibre may, for instance, end in numerous hair follicles, and each follicle is innervated by two fibres at least. The cutaneous network of each sensory spot, no matter how small, also receives branches from more than one fibre. It appears, therefore, probable that few points, and possibly only those concerned in highly organised sensations, have single private or exclusive paths to the central nervous system. Messages from a single point may travel along two or more peripheral fibres, and each fibre may carry impulses from several equipotential receptors, that is, receptors which, within certain limits, react similarly to the same stimulus. There is consequently, even in the periphery, an elaborate mechanism by which impulses excited by an external stimulus can be arranged for use of the central nervous system.

Owing to the irregular distribution of receptors in the skin, special points are more sensitive, that is, they respond to less intense stimuli, than surrounding areas. Tactile, pain and thermal spots have been mapped out, and though they are of little significance in clinical examination, in which cruder methods are usually employed, it must not be forgotten that a pinprick may be more painful in one spot than in another, and that a blunt point may excite a sensation of cold when applied to a cold spot.

The deep or proprioceptive system gives origin to impulses which subserve postural sensation, or the sense of position, the recognition of the direction, force and range of movement, the state of tension in the muscles and the perception of painless and painful pressure. The recognition of the form, size and weight of objects, and the sense of resistance by which we distinguish the hardness or softness of anything with which we come in contact, also depend mainly on impulses which arise in proprioceptive end-organs.

Disease limited to a group of end-organs of similar function, or to the fibres connected with them, would produce loss of one form of sensation only. This rarely occurs in the peripheral nervous system, but as proprioceptive afferent fibres run for a time at least with motor nerves, and those of cutaneous sensibility in sensory nerves, their functions may be involved separately by peripheral disease, the one system being affected while the other remains normal. Cutaneous dissociations do, however, occur owing to the greater overlap of fibres of adjacent nerves subserving one function than the overlap of those subserving others. When a sensory nerve is injured the area of tactile anæsthesia is usually more extensive than that in which cutaneous pain is abolished, since pain-carrying fibres of most nerves are distributed more widely than those which subserve sensibility to light touch.

Division of a nerve to any large area of skin consequently produces loss of all forms of sensation within a central area, and around it a zone of hypoæsthesia of all modes of cutaneous sensibility which increases in intensity towards the centre.

The complexity of the central pathways of sensation is incomparably greater from both the anatomical and functional points of view. Apparently every sensory impulse must traverse three superimposed sets of fibres before it can affect consciousness, and at the synapses between these sets it may be associated with related impulses conveyed by other fibres, or its components may be diverted into separate channels. The organisation of the visual system, in which this problem has been worked out more clearly by physiological methods, may serve as an illustration. Impulses which start in the rods and cones pass through a series of synapses in the retinæ before they reach the ganglion cells and fibres of the optic nerves. Within the lateral geniculate body in which they end, each of these fibres branches, and these branches terminate on several different cells. As a result each geniculate cell, which gives origin to a fibre of the optic radiation, receives messages from several optic nerve fibres, and components of the message carried by each of the latter may pass to the visual cortex by two or more geniculostriate fibres. There is consequently both multiplication of pathways and a reciprocal overlap of impulses; this overlap is probably limited to impulses of approximately the same origin and of closely related function. There is also evidence that even when they reach the cortex they follow paths broken by synapses as they ascend from its lower to its higher layers, or spread within it.

This complicated pathway is the anatomical basis of the functional organisation of visual perception. It permits both the dispersion and concentration of afferent impulses, and consequently the grouping together of those of similar or allied function. Further, at the synapses the impulses become subject to various influences which can modify them. It is probable that the pathways followed by impressions from other sense organs in their course through the central nervous system are similar.

Most external stimuli and many which act on the interior of our bodies are complex; that is, they usually excite impulses from two or more sense organs of different nature and function. A heavy contact, for instance, excites a sensation of touch as well as of pressure, and of pain if sufficiently severe; a pin-prick may be felt as touch as well as pain, and the subject may recognise the penetration of the skin by its point. Similarly, though the recognition of movement of a limb depends mainly on impulses from muscles and tendons, impressions from moving joints and from the skin around them contribute to it. It is on the multiple nature of the impressions we receive that knowledge of what is happening in our bodies and of our relations to the external world depends. Though one or other sensation excited by a stimulus may be dominant, it is the total sum of the impressions received that determine our reactions, not exclusively those of one nature or from one source only.

Some sensory impressions can be interpreted directly when related to past experiences, but others form the basis of judgments, as localisation on the surface of the body and in space, the recognition of an object in our hands, or the identification of any other stimulating object. Investigation of sensation and its disorders in disease therefore requires analysis of the impressions evoked by the stimulus into their simplest elements.

All afferent fibres reach the spinal cord through the dorsal or posterior roots. As they enter it the first sorting out and regrouping of impulses according to their function takes place. One group of fibres, which enters the dorsal column on the same side, bends cerebralwards almost immediately and runs through this column to its nuclei at the lower end of the medulla oblongata (Fig. 11). The majority of these fibres are uninterrupted, but some end in the adjacent grey matter of the dorsal horn or give collaterals to it. Since the fibres of each entering root displace medialwards those of the lower roots, in the higher segments of the cord fibres carrying impulses from the lower limbs come to lie in the dorso-median column of Goll, those from the higher parts of the body in Burdach's dorso-lateral column (Fig. 14).

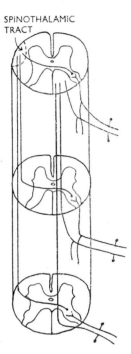

SPINOTHALAMIC TRACT

FIG. 11.

Diagram of the paths that conduct sensation through the spinal cord.

Impulses conveyed through the ipsilateral dorsal column are essential for the perception of postural sensation and appreciation of movement, recognition of the size, shape, texture and weight of objects, the localisation of cutaneous stimuli, and for two-point discrimination, the sense of resistance and probably the appreciation of vibration. These functions are not, of course, "transmitted" in the dorsal columns and clearly depend on the interpretation of data derived mainly from tactile and tension receptors.

Localisation of contacts depends on these tactile impulses conveyed through the dorsal columns. According to one view, each impulse has a specific quality or character ("local sign") which enables its point of origin to be accurately localised. It is, however, more probable that recognition of the point touched depends on the arrival in consciousness of impressions from two or more receptors, possibly through separate fibres, rather than on the specific quality of individual impulses. The wealth of end-organs in and beneath the skin, and the innervation of each by two or more fibres, permits almost unlimited combinations of impressions from them, and the special characters of these combinations furnish the material on which judgments of their origin can be based.

The remaining sensory fibres of the dorsal roots end in synapses around the cells of the dorsal horn, some at the level of their entry, others some distance above or below it, for many fibres divide into ascending and descending branches as soon as they enter the cord. This branching may be for the purpose of functional rearrangement. Each cervical, lumbar and sacral root carries afferent impulses from a long strip on an upper or lower limb, the muscles under the distal portions of which are innervated by lower segments of the cord than those under its proximal parts (Fig. 12). Anatomical economy requires a regrouping according to their origin of the exteroceptive and proprioceptive impulses concerned in reflex and other reactions; for instance, the sixth cervical root conveys sensory impulses from fingers, from the forearm and from the upper arm, while the muscles which move the fingers are innervated by the lowest cervical and first thoracic

segments and those of the upper arm by high cervical segments. The
diversion caudalwards of impulses from the hand entering by a higher
root brings them into association with others from the hand which enter
by lower roots, and permits them to terminate together in grey matter
nearer the origin of the efferent
nerves to the muscles which
move the fingers. A similar
switching through ascending
branches of impulses from the
proximal distribution of the
root brings them to the grey
matter of the segments from
which the muscles of the upper
arm receive their motor supply
(Fig. 12). Such a regrouping
of root fibres conducting sensation also seems likely from
various pathological observations; it explains the segmental disturbances produced
by lesions of a dorsal horn,
as occurs in syringomyelia, in
which the distal or the proximal portions only of several
root areas may be anæsthetic
Fig. 13).

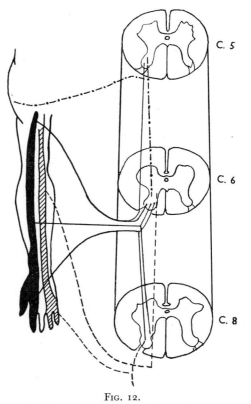

Fig. 12.

Diagram of the probable termination in the spinal
cord of afferent fibres from different portions of
the 5th, 6th and 8th cervical root areas.

The cells of the dorsal horn
around which the sensory root
fibres terminate give origin to
a second system of fibres which
crosses through the posterior
commissure to the opposite
ventro-lateral column (Fig. 11);
these are usually identified with those of the spinothalamic tract, but it is
probable that they are more diffusely arranged than those which can be
traced without interruption from the cord to the thalamus. Some probably
undergo relay in collections of grey matter along their course.

The decussating fibres of each segment displace towards the surface
of the cord those from lower segments, and consequently the path of
impulses from the arms and upper part of the trunk lies mesial to the
fibres which convey sensation from the lower limbs (Fig. 14). A lesion
advancing from the centre of the cord may therefore disturb sensation
on the upper part of the body only, or affect it earlier than that of lower
portions.

These fibres, which form a second link in the sensory chain, carry

impulses which underlie sensations of pain and temperature. The path
for thermal impulses probably lies dorsal to that which conveys painful
impressions.

There is also a path for tactile impulses in the opposite ventro-lateral
column, probably in its more ventral segment. Tickling and other affective
sensations excited by tactile stimuli depend on impressions conducted by

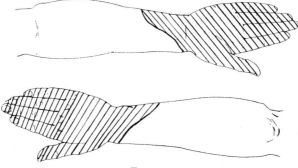

FIG. 13.

A common distribution of loss of sensation of pain and temperature on the right upper limb in syringomyelia and in other
lesions of a right dorsal horn in the lower portion of the cervical
enlargement.

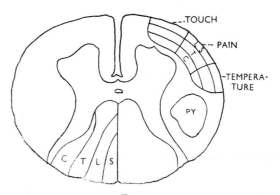

FIG. 14.

To illustrate diagramatically the positions in a cross
section of the spinal cord of the chief sensory paths. The
letters indicate the relative positions of the fibres carrying
impulses from C. the cervical, T. thoracic, L. lumbar,
S. sacral root areas (after Foerster).

these fibres. Owing to their proximity to the tract which carries pain,
sensitiveness to tickling is often lost in areas analgesic owing to spinal
lesions, though contacts can be felt as there is still a path open in the
dorsal columns to impulses that subserve it.

There are, therefore, within the spinal cord two distinct paths by
which sensory impulses from each side of the body travel towards the

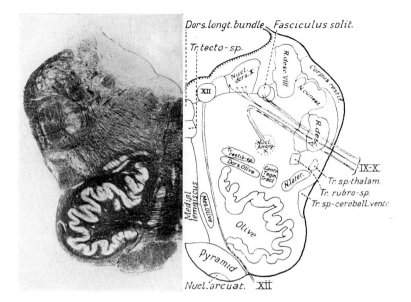

FIG. 15.

A cross-section of the medulla oblongata. The left side is stained by the
Weigert-Pal method: on the right the more important structures are outlined
and named.

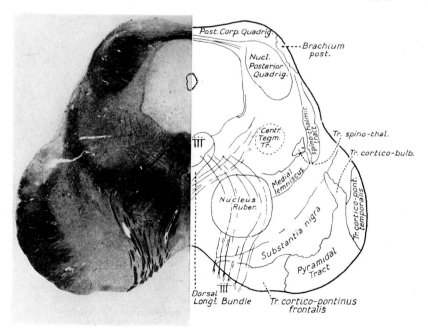

FIG. 16.

A cross-section of the midbrain. The left side is stained by the Weigert-Pal
method: on the right side some of the more important structures are outlined
and named.

brain: one in the dorsal column of the same side, the other in the opposite ventro-lateral column. Disease limited to one side of the cord above that level where the decussation of pain and temperature fibres is complete, that is, about the tenth thoracic segment, consequently produces analgesia and thermanæsthesia of the opposite side, and loss of postural sensation, accurate localisation, discrimination of compass points, recognition of shape, size and weight and appreciation of vibration on the same side. There is, however, no absolute loss of tactile sensation as there are paths on both sides of the cord through which impulses excited by contact on each side of the body can pass (Brown-Séquard Syndrome).

Within the spinal cord all impulses are collected together according to their nature. Pain, for instance, can be produced by pressure on muscles and other deep structures as well as by irritation of the skin; in the peripheral system impulses of subcutaneous origin pass along sensory fibres in the motor nerves, while those from the skin are conveyed by cutaneous nerves, but soon after reaching the cord these two groups come together and henceforth remain in company. Similarly, all impulses which contribute to recognition of posture run through the same spinal paths regardless of their origin.

At the upper end of the spinal cord the spinothalamic fibres continue to occupy the same relative position and enter the lateral portion of the medulla, but those of the dorsal columns terminate in the nuclei of Goll and Burdach. Fibres which take origin from these nuclei cross the middle line to form the medial lemniscus (Fig. 15). Above this level all sensory impulses from the limbs and trunk ascend through the opposite side of the brain-stem from that on which they entered the cord. The medulla consequently contains two anatomically separate paths for sensory impulses (Fig. 15), a lateral in which those subserving pain and termperature run, and a median which conveys those which were hitherto conducted through the opposite dorsal column of the cord. In the pons Varolii, however, the spinothalamic fibres join the lateral portion of the medial lemniscus, which has here become a broad horizontal band, and passes with it to the thalamus (Fig. 16).

Cutaneous sensory impulses from the face and head enter the medulla and pons mainly through the trigeminal and glosso-pharyngeal nerves. Some of the trigeminal fibres terminate in the main sensory trigeminal nucleus near the level of their entry; these subserve tactile sensation. A larger number turn caudalwards to form the descending trigeminal root and terminate in a nucleus which extends as far as the second cervical segment; these convey pain and thermal impulses. Fibres from the ophthalmic division extend to the caudal portion of the root, those from the mandibular branch end in the more oral part of the nucleus. Injury of the descending root consequently produces anæsthesia to pain and temperature on the same side of the face, but tactile sensation is unaffected by it. The afferent fibres of the ninth and tenth nerves also form a descending root, the fasciculus solitarius, but less is known of the arrangement of sensory impulses conveyed by these nerves from the mouth and the pharynx.

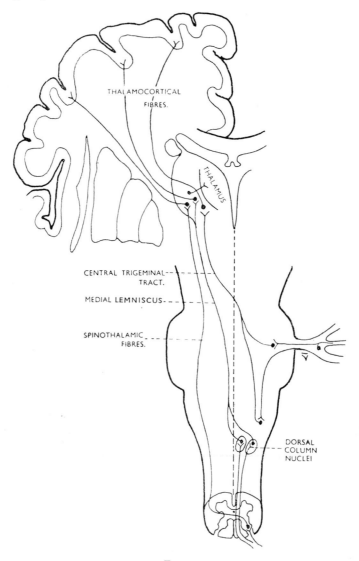

THALAMOCORTICAL FIBRES.

THALAMUS

CENTRAL TRIGEMINAL TRACT.

MEDIAL LEMNISCUS

SPINOTHALAMIC FIBRES.

DORSAL COLUMN NUCLEI

FIG. 17.
Diagram of the chief sensory paths within the central nervous system.

The secondary sensory trigeminal fibres cross the middle line and join in the medial lemniscus (Fig. 17).

The pathways by which proprioceptive impulses from the ocular and facial muscles reach the brain-stem are not fully known. Those from the latter are probably conveyed in the facial nerve, as sensation of pressure and of pain caused by pressure are not abolished by division of the trigeminal nerve.

In the mid-brain all somatic sensory impulses are conducted through the medial lemniscus, the fibres of which end in the ventro-posterior nucleus of the thalamus. Here there is a further opportunity for the rearrangement or regrouping of impulses which underlie sensation.

The thalamus is intimately connected with the cerebral cortex by both afferent and efferent fibres. Those concerned in sensation take origin in its ventral nucleus and end in the post-central gyrus, the neighbouring part of the parietal lobe, and possibly, but to a lesser extent, in the precentral gyrus. These portions of the cortex constitute the *sensory area*, that is, the reception station for all sensory impulses which reach the surface of the forebrain.

It is not, however, exclusively through the cortex that impulses conducted by the medial lemniscus excite sensation. Although it is now known that discrete cortical lesions may impair the appreciation of cutaneous pain it remains true that no matter how extensively the sensory cortex may be damaged, provided subcortical structures remain intact and are not under the influence of shock or diaschisis, sensibility to pain is never abolished, high and low degrees of temperature can be recognised, and contact and pressure can be appreciated. All crude impressions, and particularly those containing strong affective elements, can still excite sensation.

The conclusion is inevitable that certain sensations can reach consciousness directly through subcortical centres, and it is probably through the thalamus, but their accurate localisation and discrimination probably depends on the cortex.

The cortex, on the other hand, subserves all forms of discriminative sensation. It is not merely concerned in perception; it contains physiological mechanisms by which we can:

(1) Relate incoming experiences to previous sensations, and recognise similarity and differences.

(2) Become aware of the postural relations of separate portions of our bodies, and appreciate any displacement they undergo either actively or passively.

(3) Locate the sites of stimuli to the surfaces of our bodies, and distinguish betweeen one and two simultaneous contacts.

(4) Recognise the shape, size, weight, texture and consistence of objects which come in contact with us.

(5) Associate sensations of cutaneous and proprioceptive origin with other sense impressions, and particularly with those furnished by vision, and integrate them to provide the basis of our knowledge of our relations to the world around us.

Another function of the cortex is to facilitate perception of stimuli of interest at the moment, and suppress or damp down most of the multifarious impulses excited by impact of the outer world on the surface of the body and from the tissues of the body itself. The receptive centres are being continually bombarded during both waking and sleeping hours by afferent impulses, most of which are of no immediate consequence. If all reached the level of consciousness they would produce a chaotic medley which could only result in confusion. The cortex can, however, select impressions which are of interest or importance and neglect others, provided these are not too intense or too heavily endowed with affective qualities, as pain. This is mainly done by directing attention to those of interest and diverting it from others. The influence of attention may be frequently observed while testing sensation in normal persons, for if, after a series of stimuli above the normal threshold has been applied to one hand, they are suddenly, without the subject being aware of it, applied to the other hand or to a foot, they may evoke no response there till attention is awakened by their repetition.

This power of focusing attention on any portion of the body depends on the integrity of that part of the cortex of the parietal lobe in which sensation is represented. Consequently, a local defect in attention may result from a local cortical lesion.

Such a defect of local attention in the visual fields is a well-recognised phenomenon (p. 108), and it may be observed as readily during examination of tactile and other modalities of sensation. It becomes more obvious when stimuli of equal intensity are applied simultaneously to affected and normal parts, as few or no responses may be obtained from the former, though when tested separately no defect in sensation can be discovered in it. This disturbance of local attention becomes more pronounced on prolonged examination and when a patient tires or his attention is distracted. It explains other phenomena which are apt to appear when the sensory cortex is injured, as ignorance of the existence or neglect of a limb when its cortical representation is damaged (p. 154).

But in addition to facilitating perception by direction of attention, the sensory cortex also controls the response of subcortical centres to crude and affective stimuli. In this way it prevents excessive or unnecessary reactions to stimuli which might otherwise intrude in consciousness. When the cortex can no longer exert this controlling action owing to its connections with the thalamus being severed, as by such lesions as produce the "thalamic syndrome," a pin-prick, or a hot or a cold object causes excessive discomfort and an uncontrollable reaction.

Another feature of disturbances of sensation produced by lesions of the cortex is the variability and irregularity of responses to identical stimuli. At one time sensibility may appear little affected, at another apparently depressed. This is due to the lability or varying activity of cortical function. The same variability, apparently independent of external factors, is met with in the investigation of aphasia, apraxia and other highly evolved cortical functions.

As lower levels of the sensory system are readily affected by shock when its highest levels are injured, an acute cortical lesion may be accompanied by disorders of sensation that appear too widespread and intense to be attributed directly to the injury. After a cerebral hæmorrhage or thrombosis there may be for several days, or even weeks, pronounced disturbances of forms of sensibility mediated through subcortical centres. It is, for instance, not uncommon to find that even painful and thermal stimuli are not perceived on the affected side after a stroke. This is comparable to the flaccidity and depression of the reflexes in the paralysed limbs in the case of recent hemiplegia, though these reflexes and the tone of the muscles are maintained by purely spinal mechanisms. Similarly, after local epileptic seizures which begin with or include sensory phenomena there may be a temporary loss or disturbance of all forms of sensibility in the part in which the attack began, or even on the whole of that side of the body.

These distant repercussions of acute disturbance of the sensory cortex confuse the true nature of cortical sensory loss to such an extent that it can be demonstrated only by examination of cases in which disease is stationary.

Sensory Topography

The form and the distribution of disturbances of sensation which result from the lesions of the nervous system depend largely on the anatomical arrangements of the sensory paths. They are among the most important clinical signs available in the diagnosis and localisation of disease.

The spinal cord is essentially a segmental organ, each segment of which innervates the motor and sensory structures of an original segment of the body. This is still obvious in the trunk where each intercostal nerve is distributed to an area which can be marked out approximately by two transverse lines around it. When the limbs sprouted out from the early embryo they carried with them the nerves of the segments from which they developed (Fig. 18). This has obscured the original metameric arrangement, and particularly that of the motor neurons, but if on a four-footed animal, or a man placed on his hands and feet with his limbs fully extended and his arms and legs rotated outwards, a series of lines drawn at right-angles to the axis of the trunk are continued on the limbs, they outline the original dermatomes and the cutaneous distribution of the dorsal spinal roots (Fig. 19).

Division of a single root does not produce loss of sensation in the whole area of skin to which its fibres are distributed, as there is a considerable overlap of fibres from adjacent roots. The full distribution of a root on the skin is revealed by the sensation which remains when those on each side of it are divided. The areas in which sensibility to touch and pain are

F

lost then correspond closely, as the overlap of root fibres concerned with both modes is nearly equal. Such opportunities for exact observation are naturally rare and the conventional diagrams should be regarded as approximate guides making no allowance for individual variation.

In the brachial and lumbo-sacral plexuses and in the peripheral nerves there is no longer any trace of segmental arrangement of afferent fibres; a nerve may contain fibres from several roots or a proportion only of those of one. The topography of the sensory disturbances which result from a lesion of a nerve therefore differs widely from that due to division of a root. Here, too, there is a considerable but variable amount of overlap of adjacent nerves, which is considerably greater in the case of the fibres which

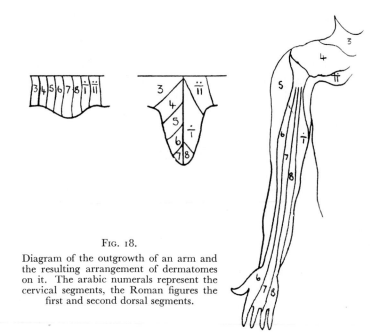

FIG. 18.

Diagram of the outgrowth of an arm and the resulting arrangement of dermatomes on it. The arabic numerals represent the cervical segments, the Roman figures the first and second dorsal segments.

conduct pain and thermal impulses than of those that carry tactile impressions. If, however, the area of skin to which the nerve is distributed is sufficiently large its division produces loss of all forms of cutaneous sensation within a portion of its area, and around this a zone of partial loss in which tactile anæsthesia is more extensive than insensibility to pain and temperature (Fig. 20). When a purely cutaneous nerve is injured, sensations from deeper structures are unimpaired as the impulses that underlie them are carried by fibres which accompany motor nerves.

The form and distribution of sensory disorders which result from disease of the spinal cord are simpler. A complete transverse lesion naturally abolishes all forms below a level which corresponds with it. The upper

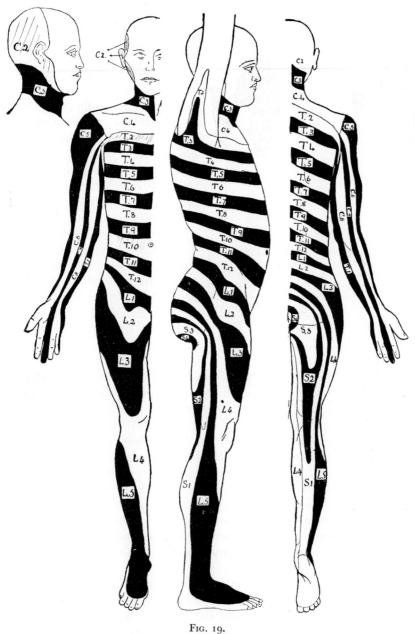

FIG. 19.

Distribution of the sensory spinal roots on the surface of the body.

margin of the anæsthesia is approximately the line between the cutaneous areas of the roots of the highest injured segment and that of the lowest intact segment.

At the upper margin of the analgesia there is frequently a narrow zone in which the patient may complain of pain, soreness, constriction or other form of discomfort. Within this zone sensibility is usually reduced; the threshold is higher, but stimuli which excite pain and many which under normal conditions do not do so, as rubbing, scraping and even simple contact if sufficiently large, are painful. This is generally a temporary phenomenon and is probably due to irritation of sensory roots, or to pathological changes of the grey matter of the cord, at the upper level of the lesion.

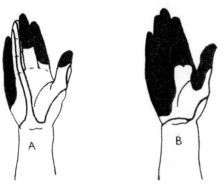

FIG. 20.

A—the average loss of sensation to touch and pin-prick on the palmar surface of the hand when an ulnar or a median nerve alone is divided; B—the loss when both ulnar and median nerves are divided. In the latter case the anæsthesia and analgesia is greater than the sum of that due to division of each nerve alone, owing to reciprocal overlapping. Insensibility to pin-prick black; tactile anæsthesia bounded by a continuous line.

Unilateral injury of the spinal cord produces those disorders of sensation included in the Brown-Séquard syndrome which has been already described, that is, analgesia and thermanæsthesia in the opposite side to a level slightly lower than that which corresponds to the lesion, and on the same side loss of those modes of sensation dependent on impulses conducted by the dorsal column. Touch escapes as there is still a path open for tactile impulses on the unaffected side.

Sensory disturbances of more irregular type and distribution result from incomplete spinal lesions. Injury of spinothalamic fibres before their decussation causes loss of sensibility to pain and temperature in zones which correspond roughly to the cutaneous distribution of the dorsal roots of the affected segments. When the disease involves them in the posterior commissure the loss is bilateral and symmetrical; when the fibres are interrupted after they pass through commissure it is contra-lateral. Such areas of loss of sensation to pain and temperature are often found in syringomyelia, in which the posterior commissure or a dorsal horn only may be involved.

As the fibres of the spinothalamic tracts are arranged in concentric layers, those conveying impressions from the lower portions of the body lying most lateral, disease invading them from without might be expected to cause first analgesia of the legs and lower part of the trunk, and only later of its higher portions (Fig. 14). This may be the explanation of the well-known fact that, when the cord is compressed, analgesia and thermanæsthesia may not extend as high as the level that corresponds to the lesion. On the other hand, when disease spreads from the centre of the cord it injures first the more mesial, and only later the lateral fibres.

This explains the fact that not uncommonly analgesia due to incomplete transverse spinal lesions does not extend over the lower sacral root areas.

Local destruction of the dorsal columns leads to loss below the corresponding level of those forms of sensation subserved by impulses conducted through them. When the injury is incomplete, different modes of sensations may suffer unequally, either because certain fibres, or certain functions of fibres, are particularly vulnerable to the pathological agent. In disseminated sclerosis, for instance, appreciation of vibration may be the only form of sensation that is affected.

Disease above the sensory decussation causes disorders of sensation on the opposite side of the trunk and on the opposite limbs. It is associated with impairment of sensation on the same side of the face and mouth when the sensory fibres of the trigeminal or glosso-pharyngeal nerves or the nuclei in which they end are involved in the lesion. As in the medulla oblongata the spinothalamic fibres are widely separated from those of the medial lemniscus derived from the dorsal column nuclei, lateral lesions of this portion of the brain-stem produce loss of sensibility to pain and temperature only, while more central lesions may disturb modes of sensation subserved by impulses carried by the dorsal columns of the cord (Fig. 15).

In the pons, however, these separate sensory paths fuse, and though the spinothalamic fibres lie for a time in the lateral margin of the fillet, lesions involving it here or in the mid-brain rarely produce dissociations of sensation.

Disease of the ventro-posterior portion of the thalamus, in which the medial lemniscus ends, causes loss or diminution of all forms of sensation on the opposite side of the body. When the anæsthesia is incomplete it may be accompanied by excessive reaction to affective stimuli, that is, those which normally excite pain or pleasure, but the threshold is raised; a light pin-prick or moderate heat or cold may not be felt, but if the intensity of the stimulus is increased it causes disproportionally severe pain or discomfort. Large or massive stimuli may be more effective in exciting such pain than smaller but more intense ones, for instances, gentle scraping with the finger nails, or a large cold surface of 22° C., causes much more discomfort than a sharp pin-prick or an ice-cold point. These disorders, often accompanied by spontaneous pains, constitute the clinical condition known as the *thalamic syndrome*. Indistinguishable symptoms may, however, arise from lesions of the sensory pathways both above and below the thalamus and the syndrome is of little localising value.

We have already seen that disease of the sensory cortex disturbs mainly discriminative sensations, that is, those by which we know the position of various parts of our bodies in space and recognise movement of them, distinguish the location of stimuli on the surface of our bodies and the sensory properties of objects which come in contact with us. These disturbances are limited to the opposite side of the body, and as there is a topographical arrangement of sensory representation in the cortex which corresponds roughly to, but is not so discrete as, motor localisation, the loss may be limited to a limb or a portion of a limb. Specific functions may also be lost or disordered in different degree, or some only may be involved; for instance, postural sensation alone may be affected, or there may be only inability to localise stimuli and distinguish two simultaneous touches from a single contact, or to recognise objects and estimate their size, weight, texture or consistence.

As might be expected sensation in the more mobile parts of the body, and particularly those employed in delicate and precise movements, are more severely affected by cortical lesions. Cortical sensory loss is therefore more prominent in the hands and feet than in the trunk and proximal parts of the limbs.

Disturbances of sensation may be limited by a sharp line or border. This occurs particularly where the sensory path is injured in the spinal cord or brain-stem. Division of a peripheral nerve usually produces loss which fades gradually into normal sensibility, but this varies from nerve to nerve, and depends partly on the severity of the injury. In polyneuritis, in which longer fibres tend to be involved earlier and more severely, the border is soft and indefinite, that is varies with the intensity of the stimulus. The true extent of the anæsthesia is revealed only by mild stimuli which approach threshold value, or by differences in the sensations evoked as compared with those from corresponding normal parts. The sensory disorders which result from cortical lesions have also soft and indefinite borders.

Hysterical or psychogenic disturbances of sensation may assume any form, but most commonly the cutaneous elements alone appear to be affected, producing failure to respond to tactile, painful and thermal stimuli. This anæsthesia is characterised by special features.

(1) Its distribution does not usually correspond with that found in organic disease of the peripheral or central nervous system. It may surround a point which had been injured, or a landmark in the body as a nipple, or it covers what the patient regards as a natural segment of a limb, appearing then as "stocking" or "glove" anæsthesia. The frequency with which its limits are determined by chance occurrences, as the level to which a limb has been uncovered, is worthy of note. If one side of the body only appears to be involved the anæsthesia frequently crosses the middle line.

(2) As a rule the borders of the anæsthesia are remarkably sharp, that is, the insensitive area adjuts immediately on the region of normal sensibility. For example, no response may be obtained to vigorous pin-pricks till a line is reached at which the patient cries out: there is usually no intermediate zone of reduced sensibility.

(3) This sharp line of demarcation is not fixed: it varies from day to day and with changing conditions of examination; for example, when a

series of stimuli are applied in succession from the normal to the anæsthetic area it may be several inches lower than when the test proceeds in the opposite direction.

(4) Disturbances are generally limited to cutaneous sensibility; postural sensation, which so commonly suffers in organic disease, is not affected, even if, as often occurs, the patient claims loss of joint position sense at the shoulder or hip. This may be easily demonstrated when, for example, a patient who presents hysterical anæsthesia of his right arm is told, "Your left arm is all right, you can move it as you like. Now I want you to bring the tip of your left index finger to the tip of your right when your eyes are closed," he succeeds at once, showing he is aware of the position in space occupied by the anæsthetic limb.

(5) The apparent loss of sensation can be modified by suggestion. If, for instance, after one leg has been found insensitive to pin-prick the patient is warned that he may feel a prick, and possibly more acutely than normal, on a small area of the sole of his foot or elsewhere, he frequently accepts the suggestion.

CHAPTER IX

Examination of Sensation

IN no sphere of clinical work is the co-operation of the patient more necessary than in the examination of sensation, as observations and conclusions drawn from it depend largely on his replies and reactions. In order to obtain reliable results it is therefore necessary to have his friendly interest and co-operation. An estimate of his mental state and of his attitude to his symptoms should precede examination, and the task presented to him and the duration of the tests should be graded to what he can accomplish without undue effort. Prolonged examinations which tire the patient and enfeeble his attention lead to confusion and error.

Children and relatively uneducated persons are often the most easy to examine as they are usually more objective and direct in their responses. Educated and introspective subjects, on the other hand, frequently confuse or mislead the observer by attempting to analyse sensations evoked by stimuli rather than by responding simply and directly to them. When a series of tests is completed the patient may, however, be asked to describe more fully the sensations they evoked.

Even normal subjects are suggestible, and many easily fall in with any lead given by the examiner. It is therefore essential that, after having explained in simple terms what is required, the examiner interposes as few questions and remarks as possible. This is particularly important in dealing with neurotic and hysterical subjects in whom disturbances of sensation and other symptoms can be easily suggested.

The patient must naturally be prevented from seeing the part under investigation. When examination is prolonged a screen between his eyes and the part under examination is preferable to closing or bandaging his eyes, as this may lead to drowsiness and failure of attention.

PAIN AND OTHER ABNORMAL SENSATIONS

Before examination is undertaken the patient should be asked to describe any abnormal sensations he has experienced. The most common of these are pain, tingling which is often described as "pins and needles," and numbness or loss of feeling. It must be realised, however, that language which has been evolved to deal with natural phenomena is often incapable of conveying the exact nature of these abnormal sensations; consequently the patient should be questioned on their nature, and a name or term which he applies to them should not be accepted at face value. Numbness, for instance, may imply a negative state, a loss of sensibility or of movement, or a positive condition, something added to the natural state.

The most common of these is *pain* which may be excited by any stimulus that threatens danger or injury to the body. The immediate reaction is reflex withdrawal of the part stimulated, but this may be followed by a more general reaction either in the form of escape or immobilisation to avoid further injury if the noxious impulses reach consciousness. Its cause may be in any organ of the body, but it is always mediated through the nervous system. The central nervous system itself is, however, insensitive to pain although the blood vessels and meninges at the base of the brain in particular are richly supplied with sensory fibres sensitive to pain.

On the other hand, pain is an almost constant symptom of affections of a sensory nerve and of a dorsal spinal root, and is then referred to their peripheral distributions. It is usually accompanied by disorders of sensation, the presence and extent of which may indicate the site of the lesion or disease. Changes in the joints of the paralysed limbs that have been allowed to lie immobile and spasms of spastic muscles are other sources of pain in nervous disease. In the rare cases in which it is due directly to affections of the central nervous system it is accompanied by characteristic disturbances of sensibility to painful stimuli.

That due to disease of viscera or of other deep structures, as joints, may be confused with pain resulting from involvement of peripheral nerve fibres when it is referred to the surface of the body. The pain of arthritis of the hip may be, for instance, mistaken for that of sciatica, and that of disease of the liver may be felt in the right shoulder or of cardiac disease in the left arm. These referred pains can be explained by a state of excessive excitability in the grey matter of the spinal cord owing to the arrival in it of a spate of abnormal impulses which do not themselves reach consciousness, but the somatic impulses which pass through it are so enhanced that they are interpreted as pain when referred to the surface or deeper structures from which they come. There may be, however, only unnatural tenderness to potentially painful stimuli in the area of reference.

While never a direct result of affections of the cerebral cortex, tactile and other impulses excited by the pain producing stimulus are referred to the spatial image of the body elaborated there, and on this the power of localising its site and forming a judgment on the nature of its exciting cause depend.

Headache is the commonest form of pain encountered in medical practice and its causes and varieties are so numerous that each case must be considered individually. The three common sites of origin of the pain are the muscles of the scalp, the arteries of the scalp and the arteries and meninges of the base of the brain and, to a lesser extent, of the convexity. Muscular pain is usually a dull constant ache often punctuated by sharper twinges and accompanied by diffuse tenderness of the scalp. Pain from the arteries of the scalp, as in migraine, is intermittent but often severe and throbbing. It is accompanied by tenderness localised around the main arteries. The headache of raised intracranial pressure is characteristically at its worst when the patient wakes in the morning. It is often absent for the remainder of the day and does not prevent sleep. It is remarkably variable from day to day and may be accompanied by other ominous symptoms such as vomiting or visual failure.

No abbreviated account can do justice to the importance of headache as a symptom or to the patience and experience needed for its proper management.

Other abnormal sensations which are commonly known as *parœsthesiœ*, may be spontaneous in the sense that there is no apparent exciting cause, though they may be influenced or modified by external agents; or they may be due to disturbances in any part of the sensory system. Similar sensations may be associated with disease of blood vessels or disorders in their autonomic innervation. No one explanation covers them all, but their distribution often indicates their cause. If they correspond to the distribution of a cutaneous nerve, this nerve is probably affected; if present only below a certain level on the trunk, they are probably due to a spinal lesion, while unilateral distribution suggests disease of the brain-stem or forebrain.

Their time relations should be ascertained, as this may indicate their origin or clinical importance; temporary or intermittent tingling of the feet, for instance, may be of little significance, but if constant it may point to a serious condition.

Finally, the patient should be questioned on the factors which relieve, intensify, or otherwise modify them.

PHYSICAL EXAMINATION

Most stimuli are composite, that is, they excite a number of elementary impressions, and it is only when these are analysed and integrated by the brain and related to previous experiences that adequate sensations result. In attempting to determine the nature and site of disease it is, however, often necessary to examine these components of complex sensations separately. Exact determination of thresholds, or measurement of acuity of sensation, is rarely required, for the task of the clinician is to detect deviations from the normal, and this can usually be done by comparison with normal parts.

Light touch, or sensations evoked by contacts so slight that they do not deform the skin materially or exert pressure on subcutaneous end-organs, can be examined by a wisp of long-fibred cotton-wool such as jewellers use. The intensity of the stimulus can be graded by varying the size of the wisp; if necessary, as in testing sensitive parts, it can be drawn out into a few fine filaments, contacts by which scarcely pass the minimal threshold for any part of the body. Camel-hair brushes are less satisfactory, as by them it is less easy to grade the intensity of the stimulus, and even the finest may exert pressure on subcutaneous tissues. It is particularly important to avoid this when testing sensation in areas where it is disturbed by injury of peripheral nerves.

Definite threshold values can be obtained by the use of von Frey's hairs, or by a suitable æsthesiometer, but this is rarely necessary. It is essential that the stimulus employed should not excite thermal impressions, as the point of a pencil or the head of a pin may when it comes into contact with a heat or cold spot.

The response is influenced by the size of the stimulus, by the pressure exerted and by the rate of its application. Accurate investigation therefore requires a uniform technique. Any movement over the surface of the skin excites additional points and reduces the threshold. Moving stimuli also tend to produce tickling and add other qualities to the sensations evoked.

Tactile sensibility varies widely in different regions of the skin; the threshold is high where it is thick or cornified, as on the soles, and much lower over hair-clad parts for the follicle of each hair is liberally supplied with nerve endings, and the hair itself, by acting as a lever, augments any pressure on its free end.

Special difficulties are encountered in examining tactile sensibility when the sensory cortex is damaged. Provided the lesion is stationary and the effects of shock have passed off, and function is not disturbed by actual or latent epileptic attacks, stimuli at the normal threshold level can be felt, but the responses of the patient to repeated contacts are irregular even when the strength of the stimulus is increased, provided it causes no pain or discomfort. This is due to defect in *local attention* to which reference has been made already. When graded tactile stimuli, all above the normal threshold, are applied, as by von Frey's hairs, it is found that the proportion of correct responses is not directly related to their intensity, but naturally the proportion increases as the strength of the stimulus is increased. In a case of left-sided parietal lesion the following results were obtained on testing the dorsum of each hand with a series of von Frey's hairs of increasing strength.

	Right Hand	*Left Hand*
21 grm./mm ^{2}		IIIIIIIIIIIIIIII
21 grm./mm ^{2}	OIIOIIIOII:: OOOIOI	
23 ,,	OOIOIOIIOII::: IIIII	
35 ,,	OIIIOIIOOIIIOIII	
70 ,,	IIIOOIIOIIIIOIII	
21 ,,		IIIIIIIIIIIIIIII

FIG. 21.

The results of a series of tests with gradually increasing stimuli. I, indicates a correct response; O, failure to perceive the contact; : a hallucinatory response. The threshold was first determined on the normal hand, and this was again examined at the end of the experiment to show that there was no failure of general attention.

As these tests show, where a lesion affects the sensory cortex an accurate threshold may not be obtainable—that is, one at which a purely tactile stimulus always excites sensation. On the other hand, when tactile sensibility is reduced but not abolished by subcortical disease all contacts can be felt if the intensity and size of the stimulus are sufficiently great.

Another confusing factor when the sensory cortex is injured is a tendency for the patient to indicate he feels a contact when he is not touched; these are known as "hallucinatory responses." As the false sensations are generally referred to a spot that had been recently stimulated they are probably due to persistence of a sensation that had not been blotted out, as it is within a short time on parts endowed with normal sensibility.

It frequently happens that though no loss of touch can be demonstrated and the threshold of tactile stimuli is not raised, a patient states contacts "feel different" from what they do in normal parts. This may be due to several causes, as defective localisation, a tendency to radiation or spread of the sensation, or to absence of tickling and other affective elements.

Pressure.—While light touch does not deform the skin and consequently excites cutaneous end-organs only, pressure affects both cutaneous and subcutaneous receptors. It can be tested by any blunt object, the temperature of which should not differ materially from that of the skin.

When the skin is anæsthetic the sensations evoked are poorly localised and the threshold is high.

The state of sensibility to moderate pressure is of relatively little importance in clinical investigation, but heavier pressure which normally produces pain or discomfort often reveals important changes.

Patients are often merely confused by being asked to analyse their sensations on being stroked with wisps of wool or blunt objects. Everyone is familiar with the sensation normally evoked by being touched with a finger and this will often reliably indicate the nature and extent of sensory loss when the conventional methods have lead to exasperation.

Cutaneous Localisation.—The accuracy of localisation varies in different parts of the body, being greater in the more sensitive parts as the face, hands and feet. The localisation of light contacts, which is usually tested, depends on tactile impulses which ascend through the dorsal columns of the cord.

It can be tested in various ways. Sometimes a patient is asked to point with his normal hand to the spot that is touched on the affected part of his body, but if owing to disturbances of postural sensation he does not know where the limb to be tested lies, this method can not be employed. He may be requested to describe the exact position of the point which is touched, but poorly educated and dull patients often find difficulty in doing so. A more satisfactory method is to require the patient to indicate the spot on a drawing or diagram of the limb (Henri's method), but many find difficulty in translating the image of the part tested to a diagram. An easier and better method is to screen the part to be investigated and place in front of the screen and within the patient's range of vision the corresponding limb of another person, or of the examiner, on which the patient can indicate with his normal hand the point that is touched.

Localisation of cutaneous stimuli is more accurate than of those which act on subcutaneous structures.

Recognition of the directions of lines drawn on the skin depends on the localisation of tactile stimuli. Ability to recognise simple figures, as letters and numerals outlined by a blunt object, is a delicate test, but as it implies identification with known figures, it may be impossible though localisation is intact.

Two-point Discrimination.—The ability to recognise whether a stimulus is single or double has been regarded as a measure of tactile sensibility, but it may be lost or seriously affected though the lightest touches can be felt. It is a specific function which may be disturbed alone by both spinal and cerebral lesions; when peripheral nerves are damaged it is always accompanied by other sensory changes.

It can be tested by a pair of compasses with blunt points; the pressure exerted should never be so great as to cause pain or discomfort. The threshold of discrimination, that is, the minimal separation of the points at which the duality of stimulus can be regularly recognised, should first be determined in the corresponding normal part. It varies enormously, from 1 mm. or less on the tip of the tongue to 6 and 7 cm. on the back. When large areas have to be examined a useful normal standard is 1 cm. on the palm and 3 cms. on the sole of the foot. It is essential that the two points of the compass should be applied simultaneously and with equal pressure, and that the replies to both single contacts and double contacts should be recorded, for in certain pathological conditions a patient may interpret one contact as two, as well as fail to recognise the double stimulus. The result of examination can be recorded by McDougall's method. The distance of the points from one another is first written down, and the responses to single contacts are recorded above a line, those to double contacts below it. The stimuli are applied at irregular intervals so that any tendency on the part of the patient to guess may be recognised (Fig. 22).

When sensation is disturbed by subcortical lesions a threshold can always be obtained, that is, the patient is able to give correct replies to a series of tests when the points are sufficiently far apart, provided he can feel the contacts; but a feature of cortical anæsthesia is a tendency to mistake one and two simultaneous touches no matter how far the latter are separated, though the proportion of correct answers naturally increases on wider separation of the points.

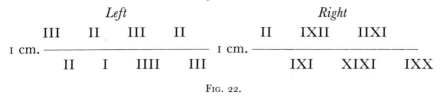

FIG. 22.

A vertical stroke indicates a correct reply, X a wrong answer. This test shows that on the left palm, which was first tested, all replies were correct, but on the right palm the patient twice confused single for double contacts, and failed to recognise the double stimulus on five occasions.

Tickling can be produced by drawing a wisp of cotton-wool or similar substance over the skin, particularly over hair-clad parts. Sensibility to it varies enormously in different regions and in different persons. In some no sensation which is recognised as tickling can be elicited, but even these persons will, when questioned, admit that a moving stimulus excites a quality of sensation in addition to, and different from, simple contact.

Tickling is often a useful test in spinal lesions; it is usually absent in analgesic areas, and it may be impossible to elicit it even in regions where there is little or no diminution of sensibility to pain. On the other hand, the reaction to tickling may be increased when responses to affective elements are exaggerated, as in the thalamic syndrome and in other conditions.

Pain.—Any noxious stimulus to the skin or subcutaneous tissues can excite pain, as a blow, a prick, a pinch, traction on hairs and extreme degrees of heat and cold, and there is still no general agreement as to how far the appreciation of pain depends on specific receptor organs.

The character of pain varies with the nature of the stimulus and with the part of the body or the organ in which it originates, but two types can be distinguished. The first, which is apparently due to excitation of receptors in the epidermis, develops quickly, as it is conducted rapidly centralwards by large fibres; it is generally described as sharp, cutting, pinching or burning, is well localised and subsides quickly. The second type, which starts in subepidermal tissues, reaches the central nervous system by finer and more slowly conducting fibres. Its onset is slower, and it tends to persist longer. It has an aching, unpleasant and less tolerable character and is less sharply localised. Variations in the nature of pain excited by a stimulus or by disease, or occurring spontaneously, may be due to the relative affection of one or other of these systems. In tabes dorsalis, for instance, the response to a pin-prick may be delayed, but the pain it causes may persist unduly long.

The sensibility of the skin to pain can be most conveniently tested by pin-prick, or preferably by the prick of a sharp needle. But even when this is employed an isolated sensation of pain cannot be obtained as the patient also feels the contact or pressure of the point, gains an idea of sharpness from its minute size, and may have, independently of the pain, a special sensation due to penetration of the epidermis. It is therefore essential to make sure that the patient replies only when he actually feels pain.

These difficulties can be, to some extent, overcome by what may be called the "covered point method." The head of the needle is held between the tip of the examiner's thumb and index finger and its stem pressed lightly against the middle finger. The point can then be withdrawn so that only the pulp of the finger touches the patient's skin, or it can be protruded so that its point penetrates the skin at the same times as the finger comes in contact with it. The patient may reply "touch" or "prick," or by "yes" when he feels the prick. When this method is employed the contact of the point when added to the pressure of the finger is less likely to be recognised, and even the sensation of penetration is reduced or blunted by the simultaneous pressure of the observer's finger. This method reduces the risk of the patient misleading the examiner by confusing contacts and pricks.

Another difficulty is that the amount of pain excited by pricks of equal intensity varies, being greater when a pain-point is touched. It is consequently advisable to take the patient's reply to a series of pricks rather than to isolated ones.

If, however, several pricks are applied in rapid succession summation may occur and exessive pain result. It must also be remembered that when pain is excited in succession in two separate parts it tends to be estimated by the patient as more severe in the place which is last stimulated. This fact must be borne in mind in comparing sensibility on corresponding parts of each side of the body; if, for example, a prick is described as sharper on the left hand when the right is first pricked, the order of the pricks should be reversed.

Normally a pin-prick can be localised accurately, but as in certain pathological conditions pain spreads or radiates from the point that is pricked, the patient should be asked to indicate where the pain is felt. In other abnormal states the perception of pain may be delayed or retarded.

Pressure pain.—Even when the skin is insensitive, pressure on deeper structures, as muscles, tendons, bones and visceral organs can cause pain. This is usually of a diffuse, unbearable or sickening character, and often produces a greater affective reaction than pin-pricks or pinching the skin. The sensitiveness of these structures can be tested best by pressure with a blunt object or by pinching muscles or tendons. Algometers which have been devised are mostly crude instruments, and special precautions are necessary to obtain a threshold to pressure pain by them.

The sensitiveness of certain visceral organs to painful pressure, as the testes and trachea, can be tested in the same manner.

"Hyperpathia."—In certain pathological conditions of both the peripheral and central nervous systems painful stimuli evoke more intense pain and a greater reaction than normal. This has been called "hyperæsthesia," or increased sensitiveness. In many cases this term is inaccurate, for, though a stimulus of sufficient intensity may cause excessive pain, the threshold is usually raised, that is, stimuli of such strength that they produce discomfort on normal parts fail to do so there; it is only when the stimulus is over the normal threshold that pain results. The term "hyperpathia," which has been proposed for this state, is consequently more suitable, but it is always preferable to describe observations than conceal them under a name.

The size of the stimulus may determine the reaction; a pin-prick may not be felt as such, but drawing the point over the surface may give excessive pain. Similarly, drawing the fingernails or a rough object over the skin, or pinching, or pressure, may cause discomfort though sensibility to pin-prick is diminished. The size of the stimulus, or more accurately the area stimulated, is the most important factor in this case too.

Thermal Sensation.—Perceptions of heat and cold are evoked only by stimuli within a small range of the thermal scale. When temperature rises above or falls below this level, it becomes a threat to the tissues, and sensation of temperatures passes into that of pain.

The recognition of heat and cold depends on the adequate stimulation of specific end-organs. As these, and particularly the "heat spots," lie relatively deep in the skin, perception is not so immediate as that of contact or pin-prick; it comes through only after a latent period, especially when small test objects are used and they are pressed but lightly on the surface of the body.

Examination of thermal sensation presents, however, many difficulties. Whether a test object is felt by the subject as hot or cold or neutral depends partly on the temperature of his skin. The neutral zone within which mild degrees of heat or cold are not perceived as such can be raised or lowered by warming or cooling it. There is consequently no exact standard of thermal sensibility. Further, as patients are prone to describe contacts which are not cool as "warm," it is necessary to understand exactly what they mean by their replies, or to intersperse neutral stimuli in a series of thermal tests.

The thermal conductivity and capacity of the test objects also influence the tests. Glass tubes containing warm or cold water are usually employed, but glass is such a poor conductor that the temperature of the surface of the tube may vary considerably from that of the water it contains, and its surface temperature is quickly modified by that of the skin. Metal tubes, preferably of silver or copper, have not this disadvantage, but unfortunately they lose heat and cold rapidly.

The response of the patient and his reaction to the stimulus is also influenced by the area of skin to which it is applied; a small object may fail to excite thermal spots; the larger it is the greater is the number of receptors which respond, and the more intense and vivid is the sensation evoked.

The essential facts for the clinician to determine are:

(1) Can the patient recognise degrees of heat and cold which can be distinguished in corresponding normal parts? It is inadvisable to use at first very hot or very cold stimuli as they may cause pain or burning, or merely discomfort if sensation is disturbed. Tubes containing water at 18° C. and 40° C. give the necessary information. Later, lower and higher temperatures can be employed, as tubes containing ice and water up to 48° C.

(2) Can he distinguish degrees of heat and degrees of cold within normal limits, as 35° C. from 40° C., or 10° C. from 20° C.? Cortical disease may disturb discrimination of degrees of temperature; it may also enlarge or widen the neutral zone, but it does not abolish thermal sensibility.

(3) If the patient states that the hot tube feels cold or vice versa the limits of the loss of thermal sensation may be outlined by drawing the tube over the skin until the patient recognises its true temperature.

Postural Sensation, or the Sense of Position.—Though a person in whom all forms of cutaneous sensibility are seriously disturbed or even abolished may be able to employ the anæsthetic limb usefully, in larger and crude movements at least, loss of postural sensation which informs us of the positions in space of all portions of our bodies and of the spatial relations of separate portions of our limbs, renders a limb practically unserviceable unless the loss is compensated by other senses, and particularly by vision.

It depends mainly on afferent impulses from muscles and joints, but cutaneous and subcutaenous impressions contribute to it. It is closely allied to the appreciation of passive movement, but it is generally advisable to examine this separately. Tests are usually limited to the limbs, but lesions involving both sides of the spinal cord or both hemispheres of the brain, may deprive the patient of accurate knowledge of positions occupied by different portions of his trunk. Unilateral loss produces no symptoms here.

Postural sensation can be tested by asking the patient, while his eyes are closed, to describe the positions into which different segments of a limb are brought, or to place the normal limb in the same relative position. To exclude sensations excited by motion of the limb it is advisable to divert his attention during the movement which brings about the new position, and to demand a reply only after an interval from its completion. If the patient is asked to look at the limb after he has described or imitated its new position, it can generally be seen by his expression if he was not accurately aware of it.

These are the most satisfactory methods when small segments of limbs, as fingers or toes, are concerned, but knowledge of position of the

G

whole limb can be tested by requiring the patient to touch or point to its extremity, as the tip of the middle finger or of the great toe, with another limb in which sensation is undisturbed.

Disorders of postural sensation are also revealed by inability to maintain steadily postures when other sense impressions, and especially vision, are excluded. If defective in both lower limbs the patient is unable to keep his balance on a small base when his eyes are closed (Romberg's sign). And if he holds both arms extended in front of him, that in which the sense of position is lacking wanders slowly from its original position; it usually droops under the influence of gravity, but it may even rise, and frequently the fingers pass through a series of irregular, purposeless postures. The subject usually fails to perceive these involuntary movements unless they are large and abrupt, and is unaware of the new position into which his limb has come, as may be seen if he attempts to touch it with his normal hand, and by his surprise when he opens his eyes.

Appreciation of passive movement is generally disturbed when there is any loss of postural sensation. It is usually sufficient to determine if the patient recognises the direction and range of a movement that he can appreciate in the normal limb, or when another limb is not available for comparison if recognition is roughly within normal standards. The only serious source of error in this test is that the patient may reply to sensations evoked by pressure of the observer's fingers on the part which is moved. In testing fingers and toes, in which disturbances are generally most obvious, this can be avoided by the observer firmly holding the digit to be moved between his finger and thumb, which should be placed on its opposite sides in the plane of the movement, or by including it within his grasp, as the additional pressure on one side cannot then be easily distinguished. Other segments of limbs should be grasped in a similar manner. Since rapid and abrupt displacements are most easily perceived, passive movements should always be carried out slowly and at a uniform rate.

If, when the movement is completed, the patient is asked to look at the part under examination, he can say if he felt the displacement which brought it into its new position and was aware of its direction.

Sense of resistance.—We can normally, even when wearing shoes, recognise whether we stand on a firm floor or on a soft carpet, on hard or on soft ground; we can distinguish whether an object with which we come into contact is hard or soft, firm or elastic; the blind man finds a safe path by his stick, and the surgeon can determine the nature of the tissue at the end of his probe; by rubbing a finger over a surface we can determine whether it is smooth or rough by the amount of resistance encountered. We obtain different impressions on moving a limb through air and through water, and can distinguish a fluid from a more viscid liquid. Recognition of these properties of objects depends largely on the resistance encountered on displacement of, or pressure against, them, either by immediate contact or by a tool or object interposed between them and the body. This sense of resistance is a composite faculty; it depends partly on touch, or rather on pressure, but mainly on the effort necessary to execute the movement, or on the opposition it meets.

Loss of sense of resistance explains many clinical symptoms, as the tabetic's complaint that he feels he is walking on clouds, and the inability of a patient with cortical anæsthesia to perceive that a solid object in his hand is anything more than something touching it. It can be tested by use of a series of objects of different consistence, but of the same size, as several pieces of rubber tubing which require different amounts of force to compress them.

Appreciation of Weight.—Defective appreciation of weight and inability to distinguish relative weights is one of the most common symptoms of disease of the sensory cortex. When the hand, which is the part usually examined, is fully supported it is really a matter of testing recognition of the pressure which the weight exerts on the surface on which it lies; when the hand is unsupported and the patient is allowed to "weigh" the object by raising and lowering it alternately, other factors come in, chiefly the appreciation of resistance to movement.

A test of the appreciation of weight by the motionless supported hand is protracted by the need to find the threshold on the normal side and is consequently of no practical importance.

With the hand unsupported and free to move two selected objects are placed in irregular sequence on each hand and the patient asked to compare their relative weights.

This is a more satisfactory test, provided the power and range of movement of the hand is not seriously reduced, for a weight tends to feel heavier to a weak limb unless its sensation is also disturbed.

It is advisable that the size or bulk of the test objects should be approximately the same; pill boxes containing different amounts of shot or lead are suitable.

Recognition of Shape.—Recognition of the shape or form of objects depends on the integration by the cortex of the forebrain of several varieties of impressions which reach it; some come from the skin, but the more important from deeper structures, for movements of the fingers over or around the object and the feeling of resistance they encounter on handling it, are even more essential than the tactile impressions which it excites. The usual test is to ask the patient to name a familiar object placed in his hand while his eyes are closed or screened, but this test implies, in the first place, recognition of its shape, and secondly, its identification, which is a more complicated process and may be impossible owing to an agnosia though no sensory disturbance is present. Sometimes, however, an object is recognised more quickly than its shape is reconstructed in the mind by synthesis of immediate impressions.

Under ordinary conditions the use of familiar objects, as coins, a key, a penknife, a pencil, is quite sufficient provided the patient does not suffer with an aphasia which makes it impossible for him to recall their names. When aphasia or agnosia prevents the patient from naming or identifying anything placed in his hand a double series of objects should be provided: one set is employed in the tests, the other is placed in front of him so that he can point to the object which he thinks corresponds to that in his hand.

If owing to paresis the patient is unable to handle freely an object, his fingers should be moved passively over it by the examiner; this usually makes it possible for him to recognise its shape unless the specific sensibility is disturbed.

Recognition of Size.—The appreciation of the absolute or relative sizes of objects is closely allied to the recognition of form. It may be tested by applying to the skin linear or flat objects of different sizes or lengths. A threshold can be obtained by using a series of objects of graded size, and determining the proportional difference at which the patient can distinguish two applied in succession.

Appreciation of Texture.—This is also a complex function, but dependent mainly on cutaneous impressions. It is, however, a useful test as it is easily disturbed, particularly by lesions involving the sensory cortex. Common materials, as tissues of linen, silk, velvet and wool may be used.

Vibration.—Disturbances in appreciation of vibration often furnish useful clinical information, though they are of little or no practical significance to the patient. They may exist alone or with disorders of other forms of sensation due to disease of the central nervous system, and particularly of the spinal cord. Appreciation is rarely influenced by injuries of single nerves, but may be lost when both cutaneous and deep afferents of several nerves are interrupted, as in polyneuritis. It is affected by cerebral lesions especially when these involve the thalamus. Acuity of perception diminishes with advancing age, especially in the lower limbs.

Perception of vibration depends on impulses from both skin and subcutaneous tissues which probably ascend through the dorsal columns of the cord, although the common association of signs of cortico-spinal tract involvement has suggested alternative routes. It has been regarded as a form of osseous or bone sensibility, but though vibrations transmitted from a tuning-fork may be conducted along bones, and though they are most readily perceived where skin and subcutaneous tissues are firmly compressed between the base of the fork and underlying bone, they can be felt when the fork is applied to a fold of skin raised from the skeleton.

In testing sensibility to vibration a heavy tuning-fork should be employed, as C° of 128 vibrations per second. Various devices have been employed to measure sensibility, but comparison with a corresponding normal part, of either the patient or the observer, is usually sufficient. The base of the fork is usually placed over superficial bones, but vibrations can be equally well felt when it rests on other firm tissues, as the palm or sole. As the thorax acts as a resonator local loss cannot be demonstrated by placing the fork on a rib; it is therefore advisable when applying the test to the trunk to bring the fork into contact with folds of skin raised from the chest. When used in this way the test is often helpful in determining the extent of sensory disturbances due to spinal lesions.

In ordinary clinical examination it is rarely necessary to investigate the state of all these forms of sensation, or employ all the tests described here; experience soon teaches the student which are essential in any type of case he may meet. When a peripheral nerve is injured the state of light touch and pin-prick are most important; when the spinal cord is affected, sensibility to pin-prick and thermal stimuli is more frequently involved than touch, and loss of postural sensation and the appreciation of vibration are often pronounced. Tactile sensibility is relatively more affected by lesions of the brain-stem. Predominant loss of the discriminative elements characterises cortical disease, particularly disturbances in the recognition of posture and form, the localisation of cutaneous stimuli, the distinction of double from single contacts, and the appreciation of weight and texture, but any of these qualities may escape.

CHAPTER X

Reflexes

THE importance of reflexes in clinical neurology is, in the first place, due to the fact that they are largely independent of co-operation by the patient, and consequently more objective evidence than many other physical signs; and, in the second place, alterations in their intensity or character are frequently the most delicate indications we possess of disturbance of function. Although reflexes are regarded as the simplest and most stable of nervous activities, the ease with which they can be elicited, and even their presence, depend on many factors and on the conditions under which they are tested. These will be discussed in the following paragraphs.

By a reflex is generally understood a response, usually in the form of movement, to a peripheral stimulus without the intervention of consciousness, but the term has been extended so widely that this definition is insufficient: in cerebral reflexes and in conditioned reflexes, perception and processes involving some degree at least of consciousness are involved.

Reflexes may be, according to their nature, placed in various categories.

1. *Tendon Jerks* (Deep Reflexes) are responses of muscles by contraction to sudden stretch imposed on them.

2. *Cutaneous Reflexes* (Superficial Reflexes) are immediate reactions to stimuli to the surface of the body, but analogous reactions may be evoked by stimuli to other sensory surfaces, as contraction of a pupil to light falling on the retina, involuntary movement of the head to a sound, and secretion of saliva when a bitter substance is introduced into the mouth.

3. *Postural Reflexes* which control or correct postures of the body and its limbs in response to impulses (proprioceptive) from deeper structures, especially from muscles and the labyrinths.

4. *Cerebral Reflexes*, in which response to an adequate stimulus requires the intervention of perception.

5. *Visceral Reflexes.*—These are concerned in the activities of the visceral organs. In clinical neurology use is made only of those which control the functions of the pharynx, bladder and rectum. These will be described in the chapters devoted to these organs.

6. *Condition Reflexes* which have, however, little significance in clinical work.

7. *Autonomic Reflexes*, especially those concerned in vasomotor control and pilomotor activity.

STRETCH REFLEXES

The importance of the stretch reflex in the control of movement and posture was described in Chapter V. The phasic stretch reflexes, the response to rapid stretch, are of immense value to the clinician.

The *knee jerk* may be taken as a typical example and used to illustrate the technique of elicitation, the modifying factors and the significance of deviations from the normal.

The knee jerk is usually elicited by a sharp blow or tap on the patellar tendon where it bridges the gap between the patella, to which the extensors of the knee are attached, and the front of the tibia. Depression of the tendon into this gap draws down the patella and suddenly stretches the

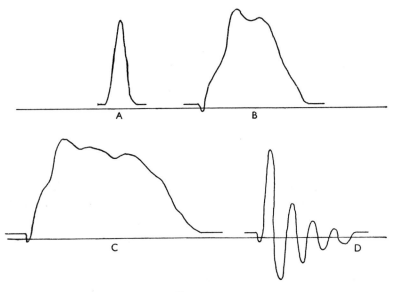

FIG. 23.

A—tracing of a simple muscle twitch, B—of a normal knee jerk, C—of a knee jerk in a spastic limb, D—of a pendular knee jerk from a patient with an acute cerebellar lesion.

extensor muscles of the knee, which respond by shortening and extending the knee joint. If the patella is immobile owing to ankylosis, or if the tendon is so slack that its depression does not displace the patella, no reflex is obtainable. A sharp blow on the upper edge of the patella is equally effective, provided it stretches the quadriceps, and if reflex excitability is high a jerk can be elicited by a tap on the tibia, or even on the dorsum of the foot, provided the limb is in such a position that the blow flexes passively the knee and thus stretches its extensor muscles. It is not the blow on the bone or stimulation of the tissues which cover it which evoke the reflex: only those manipulations are effective which stretch the muscle.

It is obvious, therefore, that such terms as "reflexogenous zones" are inapplicable to stretch reflexes, though the ease with which they can be elicited by different manœuvres may be a measure of their activity.

The knee jerk consists of a sudden twitch-like contraction of the muscle, to which is added a short tonic contraction that gradually subsides and allows the extended leg to fall. A tracing of the contracting muscle shows these two components, an abrupt rising of the tracing, and a short plateau or hump before the muscle relaxes (Fig. 23). Modifications in these components characterise the knee jerk in certain normal and pathological conditions. When reflex excitability is high the contraction is abrupt and strong, the amplitude of the jerk is large, and it can be elicited by a smaller stimulus. If the tone of the quadriceps is increased, the tonic phase is more pronounced and of longer duration, and the leg is consequently held extended for a time, and falls slowly and often irregularly owing to the occurrence of secondary contractions that are also due to tension on the extensor muscles (Fig. 23).

The response to a tap on the patellar tendon depends on several factors. In the first place, the direction of the blow is important: when it is directed upwards on the lower border of the patella a jerk may not be elicited, as such a blow may not stretch the quadriceps; while a glancing blow in the downward direction which tends to draw the patella down as well as depress its tendon evokes a brisk response.

The state of tension in the quadriceps muscle is more important. Some degree of reflex tone is essential, but the resting length of the muscle plays a part too. It may be impossible to obtain a jerk if the quadriceps is fully extended by maximal flexion of the knee, or shortened by its full extension. This is more obvious in the case of the ankle jerk and the stretch reflexes of the arms. For this reason the knee jerk is usually tested when the knee is semi-flexed and the leg hangs unsupported, but it can be obtained with equal ease when the patient lies on his side, or if, while he is supine, the knee is raised by the observer's hand placed behind it so that its extensor muscles are on slight tension.

As the tone of the quadriceps is relaxed reciprocally when the hamstring muscles contract either reflexly or voluntarily, the jerk may be unobtainable when the leg is in flexor spasm, or while the subject attempts to flex the knee. This is the most common source of error when a normal jerk cannot be demonstrated. On the other hand, a general increase of tension, as in emotional states and on strong muscular effort of some other part of the body, augments the response. A knee jerk absent on normal testing may appear on reinforcement. This is usually effected by Jendrassik's manœuvre of a strong hand grasp or powerful effort of the arms against resistance. This probably acts by increasing the sensitivity of the receptor organs in the muscle spindles by increased fusimotor activity. A local increase of tension in the quadriceps is equally effective: this can be obtained by making the subject extend his lower limb gently against a resistance; in fact, the most effective method of reinforcement is to make him press the anterior part of his sole against the observer's hand, against the floor or other object while the jerk is being tested. This method has the additional advantage that extension of the limb prevents voluntary contraction of the hamstring muscles and consequent reciprocal relaxation of the extensors of the knee.

The activity of the reflex is estimated by the vigour of the response, its duration and by the range of movement of the leg. When, however, reflex excitability is high the range of the jerk may be restricted by reflex contraction of the opposing flexors of the knee, owing to the abrupt stretch to which they are exposed by extension of the joint.

CLONUS.—When a muscle in a state of high reflex excitability is exposed to continuous stretch it may contract intermittently, a series of reflexes develop which produce rhythmical movements, regular in time and amplitude and at a rate of about eight per second. Clonus is most easily elicited at the ankle by passively dorsiflexing the foot and maintaining pressure on the sole, but knee clonus can be demonstrated by drawing the patella downwards, or by abruptly raising the knee while the limb is extended so that the weight of the leg suddenly stretches the quadriceps. A series of rhythmical reflex contractions of this and of other muscles in the form of clonus may occur in spastic limbs when they are suddenly stretched by cutaneous or proprioceptive reflexes, each beat is caused by renewed stretching of the muscle after relaxation of its previous contraction. A few beats of ankle clonus can often be found in tense but otherwise normal patients. In spastic limbs clonus is often inexhaustible, persisting for as long as stretch is maintained, and may be present in other muscle groups such as the flexors of the fingers.

To and fro movements at a joint simulating a clonus may occur in hysterical and other neurotic states. They can readily be distinguished from true clonus by the obvious alternating contractions of prime movers and their antagonists and by the fact that they are not regularly induced by stretch or inhibited by passive shortening of the muscle.

The chief pathological factor that depresses reflexes is interference in the functional activity of the reflex arcs on which the tone of the muscles also depends. Disturbances in the afferent or efferent limbs of the arc, or of the spinal reflex centre, so mild that they cause no demonstrable defect in motion or sensation, suffice to abolish or depress stretch reflexes. Their loss is consequently a delicate indication of lack of functional integrity, and usually of the presence of an anatomical lesion.

Occasionally, however, these reflexes are unobtainable though the reflex arc is structurally intact, as in states of spinal shock, or when the tone of the muscles concerned in the response is inhibited by another reflex or by contraction of their antagonists. In "paraplegia-in-flexion," for instance, the knee jerks may be unobtainable, and they may be absent or difficult to elicit in the generalised rigidity of advanced Parkinsonism. Knee jerks also disappear in deep sleep, and are sometimes unobtainable in fevers, though there may be no evidence of nervous disorder.

Pathological exaggeration of the tendon jerks is usually associated with increase of tone in the contracting muscles, and is therefore present in spastic states in which spinal reflex mechanisms are released from control of higher nervous levels. It has been assumed that this inhibiting control is exerted through the pyramidal tracts, but in addition to certain physiological evidence the fact that increase of the jerks may be greatly out of proportion to other evidence of pyramidal disease suggest that loss of corticospinal impulses is not wholly responsible. There is evidence that it may be due to lack of impulses carried by the vestibulospinal tracts; they are usually most exaggerated when the ventro-lateral columns of the cord which contain these tracts are injured.

The knee jerks, and the same is true of other stretch reflexes, may be also pathologically brisk when the tone of the opposing muscles is low; as when, in the case of the knee jerk, a flaccid palsy of the hamstring muscles exists. This permits a fuller swing of the leg, and it also abolishes or diminishes the reciprocal inhibition of the quadriceps from the flexors of the knee. In states of muscular hypotonia, as in cerebellar disease, the swing of the leg may be more ample than normal owing to the toneless- ness of the knee flexors: partly owing to this, partly to lack of tonic pro- longation of the contraction, the leg may continue to swing as a pendulum —the pendular reflex (Fig. 23).

Other pathological alterations in these reflexes occur in various dis- cases. In chorea minor, and occasionally in states of low muscle tone, the first tap on the patellar tendon may fail to evoke a knee-jerk, but on repeated tapping a brisk response may be obtained. The early taps are subliminal stimuli which summate to give a normal reflex. In chorea a characteristic *sustained knee jerk* is sometimes obtained, the leg remaining extended owing to prolonged contraction of the quadriceps.

The constancy of the knee jerk in normal persons, and the ease with which it can be elicited, are responsible for the importance rightly attached to it in clinical work. Although individuals are occasionally met in whom these reflexes have been absent for years without a history of past or evi- dence of present illness, they are so few that their absence should always be regarded as a sign of disease. Unusual briskness, on the other hand, is not necessarily pathological, as it occurs when the tension of the quad- riceps is high, as in emotional states, in hysteria, and when a moderate degree of voluntary contraction is present in the muscles.

Under suitable conditions a reflex contraction of almost every muscle can be obtained by stretching it abruptly, and a large number of such phasic stretch reflexes have been described, but relatively few are made use of in routine clinical work. Others may be helpful in the localisation of spinal and other lesions. These reflexes are better designated by the muscle which responds or the movement produced than eponymously. The general rule is that the resulting movement is in a direction opposite to that of the blow which elicits it. Some are easily excited by any adequate stimulus, others only when reflex irritability is high, as in spastic states.

The following are examples of stretch reflexes which can be easily demonstrated.

When the cheek is retracted by a spatula in the angle of the mouth, a sharp tap by a percussion hammer on the spatula excites contraction of the muscles which are stretched by the tap. A tap in the outward direction on the outer margin of the orbit results in a contraction of the orbicularis palpebrarum and closure of the lids. A downward blow on the point of the shoulder may produce elevation of the whole limb, and one on the angle of the scapula, adduction of the scapula and of the arm. When the inner condyle of the humerus is percussed sharply, the adductors of the arm contract and draw it towards the side.

In the trunk stretch reflexes are less easily demonstrated, but when a finger resting on the front of the abdomen is tapped, the underlying muscles may be felt to contract, provided the abdominal wall is not too lax, or this can be excited by a sharp blow near their insertion on the costal margins.

Stretch reflexes are more easily elicited in the lower limbs. The blow of a percussion hammer on the internal condyle of the femur, or, if reflex excitability is high, on the inner side of any segment of the limb, causes adduction of the thigh, and often of the opposite thigh too, as contraction of the ipsilateral muscles exerts a slight but adequate strain on the contralateral adductors. When a finger placed on the tendon of one of the hamstrings is tapped the corresponding muscle contracts.

The reflexes usually employed in clinical examination deserve further notice and description of the most suitable methods of eliciting them. The knee-jerk has been already dealt with as a type of these reflexes.

The Ankle Jerk is a brisk contraction of the extensors of the ankle and plantar extension of the foot in response to a tap on the tendo Achillis. It is most easily obtained when the knee is partly flexed and the foot dorsiflexed by the examiner to such an extent as to exert slight tension on the muscles of the calf. When the reflex is brisk the contraction of the gastrocnemius may also flex the knee. If exaggerated the initial jerk may be followed by *ankle clonus*, provided passive stretch on the calf muscles is maintained.

The ankle jerk is not so constant in normal persons as the knee jerk; it may be difficult to demonstrate in children, and is often absent in aged subjects. Permanent absence may follow sciatica or peripheral neuritis, or may be temporarily due to œdema of the leg.

ARM JERKS.—Those usually tested involve movement at the elbow joint.

The Flexor Jerk is an abrupt contraction of the flexors of the elbow—biceps, brachialis anticus and brachio-radialis—when these are stretched by a blow on the forearm which tends to extend the elbow. It is most satisfactorily elicited by a tap on the lower end of the radius while the elbow is flexed to approximately a right-angle and semi-pronated; the examiner should at the same time exert slight tension on the flexor muscles of the elbow by extensorward traction. When the efferent limb of the reflex arc to one of the muscles is interrupted, the others suffice to produce the reflex; for instance, the brachio-radialis alone may flex the elbow when the biceps and brachialis anticus are palsied or toneless. If, in addition, the brachio-radialis fails to respond, the elbow may be flexed by the long flexors of the fingers, which are accessory flexors of the elbow when the arm is pronated; then flexion of the fingers naturally occurs too.

The reflex excitability of the individual flexors may be tested separately; if a finger placed on the tendon of the biceps is tapped, this muscle only contracts as it alone is stretched. It is usual to refer to the *supinator jerk* excited by a tap on the radius and to the *biceps jerk* elicited from that muscle directly.

In states of reflex hyperexcitability the response may spread beyond those muscles obviously stretched; in particular the fingers may flex. If there is a lesion of the sixth cervical roots or segment the normal flexor response will be absent but the blow from the tendon hammer may be sufficient to cause minute stretch of the finger flexors which then contract in isolation. This is known as *inversion* of the biceps or supinator jerk.

The Extensor Jerk of the Forearm (Triceps Reflex) is an extension of the forearm elicited by a sharp tap on the tendon of the triceps when the elbow is flexed to approximately a right-angle. The triceps is the only muscle concerned in this reflex.

When the seventh and eighth cervical segments or roots are injured, a blow on the tendon of the triceps or on the olecranon may cause flexion instead of extension of the forearm: this is known as *inversion of the triceps reflex*. It has been attributed to over-excitability of the flexor jerk, but a more probable explanation is that the blow extends the joint passively, though to a minimal extent, and consequently stretches its flexors.

Pronator Jerk.—When the forearm is in semi-pronation a glancing blow on the dorsal aspect of the lower end of the ulna by causing slight supination stretches the pronators and excites a reflex contraction of them and pronation of the forearm.

Finger Jerk.—This reflex cannot always be elicited in normal persons, but it is a valuable indication of disease when it is asymmetrical or present on the one side only. It is best demonstrated by the observer placing his fingers across the palmar aspects of the tips of the patient's fingers while they are extended at the metacarpo-phalangeal and flexed at the inter-phalangeal joints, and exerting slight pressure in the direction of extension of the distal joints, which must, however, remain in flexion; a tap on his own fingers will then cause flexion of the patient's fingers and thumb owing to reflex contraction of their long flexors.

Jaw Jerk.—A tap on the chin when the teeth are separated and the jaw relaxed, occasionally in normal persons and in certain pathological conditions, leads to closure of the jaw. As this is effected by contraction of bilaterally acting muscles unilateral lesions have little influence on it. Only exaggeration of the jaw jerk is of clinical significance. The afferent and efferent limbs of the reflex arc of this reflex run through the sensory and motor roots of the trigeminal nerve.

SUPERFICIAL REFLEXES

These reflexes are excited by stimuli acting on the surface of the body, either on the skin (cutaneous reflexes) or the mucous membranes. Adequate stimuli are not so specific as in the case of the stretch reflexes; a gentle touch, a stroke, tickling, a pin prick, hot or cold contacts and other noxious or harmless stimuli may be effective. Further, the ease with which they can be elicited varies considerably, partly owing to local conditions, as the temperature and state of the skin.

The Abdominal Reflexes are typical examples. A stroke with a blunt object, a prick and sometimes even a touch on one side of the abdomen excites contraction of the underlying muscles and deviation of the midline towards the point that is stimulated. The reflex centre of the upper abdominal, or epigastric, reflex, which is evoked by stimulation of the skin above the level of the umbilicus, lies in the seventh to ninth thoracic segments, that of the lower reflex in the tenth and eleventh segments. The epigastric reflex is best elicited by an oblique stroke from without inwards close to and roughly parallel with the costal margin. This results in deviation of the umbilicus and of the middle line towards the stimulus. Similarly, a stroke on a lower segment of the abdominal wall draws the umbilicus downwards and towards the same side. If the reflexes are feebler or lost on one side a stroke along the middle line of the abdomen may draw it towards the other side.

In testing these reflexes it is important that the stimulus should not stretch the underlying muscles, for if these are spastic they may contract to sudden stretch and simulate a true cutaneous reflex.

These reflexes can be obtained in most normal persons unless the muscles of the abdominal wall are lax and feeble, as in some multiparæ and in advanced age. They often disappear in acute abdominal disease. When in obese subjects it is not possible to observe the movement it can usually be felt by fingers pressed lightly on the abdominal wall.

The abdominal reflexes have a polysynaptic arc in which the pyramidal tract appears to form a link as the reflexes disappear in affections of the upper motor neurons, and are, in fact, the most delicate sign we possess of their disorder; their diminution or absence is often the earliest indication of a progressive lesion involving the pyramidal motor system in the brain or spinal cord. In very slight disturbances of corticospinal function there may be only a tendency for the reflexes to tire or disappear on repeated stimulation of the skin. In peripheral palsies of the abdominal wall they also disappear. As they are occasionally unobtainable though no nervous disease exists, asymmetry or unequality of them is the essential fact of clinical significance.

Though so frequently abolished by pyramidal disease acquired in adolescent or adult life, these reflexes can often be obtained in the presence of corticospinal palsies dating from childhood, as in infantile hemiplegia and diplegia, and they may persist in the early stages of certain systemic degenerations, as *motor neuron disease*, though other signs of spastic paresis are present.

Occasionally, and chiefly in spastic states, a reflex retraction of the antero-lateral wall of the abdomen at about the level of the umbilicus is evoked by a firmer stimulus than is usually necessary to excite a true abdominal reflex. It is often bilateral, does not deviate the midline of the abdomen towards the stimulus, and may be associated with a flexion reflex of the lower limbs.

Since these reflexes are segmental, that is, it is those muscles or portions of muscles which are innervated by the same segments of the cord that receives the cutaneous impressions that contract most vigorously, they are of great value in the localisation of lesions in the lower half of the thoracic cord. If, for instance, the ninth thoracic segment is involved no response is obtained to a series of stimuli from below upwards, or the response is subnormal in intensity or tires easily, till the level of the umbilicus is reached; then the muscles innervated from the segment next above that which is affected react normally.

To elicit these reflexes it is important that the abdominal wall is relaxed. When it is difficult to obtain sufficient relaxation, the stimulus should be applied only at the end of expiration.

Cremasteric Reflex.—Stroking, pinching or pricking the skin of the upper and internal aspect of the thigh excites contraction of the cremaster muscle and elevation of the testicle on the same side. It should be distinguished from contraction of the dartos muscle which draws up the same side of the scrotum. The cremasteric reflex is of little practical importance except in the localisation of lesions involving the upper lumbar segments in which its centre lies, or their afferent or efferent fibres. It often is abolished by lesions of the corticospinal tracts.

Plantar Reflex.—Stimulation of the sole by stroking with a blunt object or by prick leads to immediate withdrawal of the limb by flexion at the hip and knee, dorsiflexion of the ankle and flexion of the toes. This is the ordinary "withdrawal reflex" from an unpleasant or noxious stimulus which can be evoked in both normal and pathological conditions.

Portions of this reflex, and particularly the movements of the toes, have acquired a pre-eminent importance in clinical neurology, as when the functions of the pyramidal system are disturbed the response assumes a characteristic pattern.

On stroking or pricking the normal sole the great toe at once flexes and the other toes flex and adduct. This is the normal *"flexor response."* When, however, the conduction of certain cerebral impulses through the pyramidal tract is interfered with or blocked by any form of disease, or when the corticospinal system is functionally deranged as by shock, or not fully developed, as in infancy, the same stimulus produces slow, forcible but often intermittent extension of the great toe at the metatarso-phalangeal joint: this is the *"extensor response"* or Babinski's sign. It is often accompanied by extension and abduction of the other toes which spread out as the rays of a fan (*signe de l'éventail*), and by contraction of other muscles, especially of the hamstrings and of the tensor fasciæ femoris. The essential feature of this abnormal response is, however, extension of the great toe.

The plantar reflex is best tested by stroking the sole slowly with a blunt object from the heel towards the toes. Unless the corticospinal disturbance is considerable the response depends, however, on the conditions under which it is tested. In the first place, stimulation of the inner margin of the sole may give a flexor or indefinite response, though from the outer margin a characteristic extensor reflex can be obtained. Further, the posture of the limb may influence the response; though it may assume the extensor type when the limb is fully extended, the response may tend towards the flexor type when the hip and particularly the knee are partly flexed. As slow extension of the great toe is invariably an abnormal sign, no matter how elicited, the plantar reflex should therefore always be tested by stroking the outer side of the sole with the limb fully extended.

A doubtful response may sometimes be made to assume the characteristic extensor pattern by passively over-extending the knee by firm pressure on the lower end of the thigh as the patient lies on his back.

The plantar reflex is so important that the clinician should never be satisfied with failure to elicit it by ordinary means. Only a severe degree of anæsthesia of the sole, or interruption of the reflex arc which passes through the first sacral segment, abolishes it, but it is frequently difficult to elicit when the foot is cold; then warming or vigorously rubbing the sole before testing usually makes it possible to obtain a response. Ankylosis of the metatarso-phalangeal joint may, however, preclude reflex flexion or extension.

Occasionally the sole is so sensitive that voluntary withdrawal and irregular movements of the toes obscure the reflex. This difficulty can usually be overcome by drawing a blunt object, even the pad of a finger, firmly but slowly along the sole, or by stimulating the outer margin of the foot rather than the sole.

Other methods of testing the great toe reflex have been recommended, as drawing a finger firmly downwards along the outer border of the tibia (Oppenheim), or kneading or pinching the calf muscles, but they rarely add usefully to the information obtainable by plantar stimulation.

When in a case of spastic paraplegia the sole of one foot is stimulated the withdrawal of this limb is followed by a slowly developing extension of all segments, including the great toe, of the opposite limb: this produces a *crossed extensor response* of the great toe. While the ipsilateral extensor toe reflex is part of a withdrawal reflex, the crossed reflex is a component of a contralateral extensor reaction.

An extensor response is, with few exceptions, always evidence of affection of the corticospinal system, and usually appears with the slightest disturbance of its function. The reflex, however, assumes the extensor pattern in the first year or so of infancy, during deep sleep and in coma, under the influence of certain poisons, as by the barbiturates, and in the functional exhaustion that follows an epileptic seizure. When the flexors of the toes, and particularly the short flexors, are paralysed, the great toe may respond by the only movement possible to it, that is, extension.

Mass Reflex.—In cases of severe transverse lesions of the spinal cord noxious stimuli to the lower limbs, and occasionally to any part of the body below the level of the lesion, may excite, in addition to flexion of the legs, flexor spasms of the abdominal muscles, evacuation of the bladder and rectum and sweating on the paralysed parts.

Dorsiflexion Reflex of the Foot.—When the functions of one pyramidal tract are disturbed pinching or pricking the skin on the dorsum of the foot may cause dorsiflexion of the ankle, which never occurs in the absence of corticospinal disease.

Corneal Reflex.—A light touch on the cornea with a smooth, blunt object or a fine wisp of cotton-wool leads to abrupt closure of both eyes by contraction of the orbicularis muscle of the lids. Disturbances in its reflex arc, in which the fifth and seventh cranial nerves are concerned, abolish the reflex, but if only the seventh nerve is damaged on the side tested the opposite eye will still close in response to the stimulus.

Palatal Reflex.—A contact on one side of the soft palate causes its elevation, which is usually greater on the side stimulated, and is often accompanied by its deviation to this side.

The Pharyngeal Reflex, which initiates deglutition, may be excited by a firm touch with a blunt or sharp object on one side of the pharynx. It consists in contraction of the ipsilateral muscles, often accompanied by retraction of the tongue and by retching.

The Grasp Reflex may be included among the superficial reflexes, though it is mainly dependent on proprioceptive stimuli, especially tension on the flexor tendons of the fingers. The fact that it may be obtained when the skin of the palm is anaesthetic shows that cutaneous stimuli are not essential.

It should therefore be regarded as a tonic reflex of proprioceptive origin. Since it is present during the first few months of life it can be looked upon as an innate reflex which in later life is suppressed by cerebral centres, and may reappear when these are damaged. In its characteristic form it is found only with lesions of the opposite frontal lobe of the brain, but a somewhat similar response may be obtained in both hands in stuporose or dull patients with increased intracranial pressure. When present on one side only it is a sign of localising value.

It is elicited by a firm stroke in the radialward direction across the palmar surfaces of the fingers and the adjacent palm. All the fingers flex and grasp the object, but it differs from an ordinary grasp by the fact that the thumb is usually fully extended at its interphalangeal joint and adducted, so that the main force is exerted between it and the index finger. An attempt to withdraw the object radialwards increases the force of the grasp, but pressing it ulnarwards, that is, further into the hand, tends to relax it. The grasp persists as long as the stimulating object remains in the hand, especially if the observer exerts a slight pull on it. While the reflex is present the patient may be unable to open his hand voluntarily while it contains an object, though able to do so when it is empty. It cannot be obtained when the corticospinal system is seriously affected.

The grasp reflex can be most satisfactorily tested by the examiner using two or three of his fingers as the stimulating object, but a moving contact with any object, even bedclothes, may excite it.

Reflex Groping.—In patients who present the grasp reflex slowly repeated contacts on the fingers or palm may excite movements of the hand in the direction from which the contacts came; the patient appears to follow or grope towards the object which touched him, the object seems to act as a magnet which attracts the affected hand.

Postural Reflexes

Experiments on animals, particularly after removal of the forebrain and, in some instances, of deeper structures, have shown that the essential factors in the maintenance and re-establishment of postures or attitudes of the body as a whole and of its different parts are a series of proprioceptive reflexes from the muscles and their tendons, and from the labyrinths.

The importance of the reflex control of muscular contraction in this function has already been emphasised and this may be widely influenced by afferent impulses from the labyrinth and from the muscles of the neck. Such reflexes play an important part in maintaining the correct orientation of the body in space. The activity of these reflexes is difficult to demonstrate in intact animals, and particularly in man, and at present their importance in clinical medicine is slight, but they become apparent in certain release states. In spastic hemiplegia, for instance, passive rotation of the head to one side increases extensor tone in the limbs of the side to which the chin points and flexes the opposite arm (p. 128).

H

CONDITIONED REFLEXES

The investigation of the phenomena to which Pavlov has applied this term has thrown considerable light on the functional activity of the intact nervous system; they depend on the integrity of the cerebral cortex. They have shown, for example, the laws which control habit formation and the nature of certain aspects of inhibition, especially that in which the higher centres are concerned.

The essential feature of a conditioned reflex is that when a cerebral reflex is combined with an indifferent stimulus the latter may, when repeated alone, evoke the response. For instance, if the secretion of saliva excited by the sight of food is combined repeatedly at short intervals with a musical note, the latter alone may excite salivation.

Conditioned reflexes have at present little application in clinical neurology.

CEREBRAL REFLEXES

This term may be applied to a large series of responses to stimuli which also excite perception or sensation, and in which the participation of the cerebral cortex is necessary. Some of these are abolished by cortical lesions, others become obvious only when certain cortical functions are disturbed.

The majority of these reflexes are excited by retinal stimuli, in fact in man all reflexes of retinal origin are, with the exception of the pupillary reflexes, in this sense cerebral.

Blink Reflex.—The abrupt and unexpected approach of an object towards the eyes causes blinking or closure of the lids. That this is not a voluntary reaction is shown by the fact that the response to a threat from one side may be abolished by a small lesion of the opposite parietal cortex, though vision and the innervation of the muscles concerned are intact. The blink reflex is consequently at times useful in the localisation of cortical lesions.

Fixation Reflex.—The initiation of fixation of the eyes on an object is usually volitional, but it is reinforced and maintained by a reflex which tends to keep the eyes directed on the object in central vision. The afferent path carries retinal impulses from the region of the maculæ to the visual cortex, the efferent impulses probably run directly from the occipital lobe to the mid-brain.

This reflex may become dominant when the voluntary movements of the eyes are impaired; then the patient may have difficulty in disengaging his vision from any point on which it is directed.

The Fusion Reflex determines the accurate directing of the eyes so that the images of the object in attention fall on corresponding points of the two retinæ. It frequently fails in asthenic or toxic states with the result that vision is not distinct; the patient may complain that in reading the letters of the print run into one another. It is often defective when one or more of the external ocular muscles is paretic; the images of objects then appear blurred, but double vision may not be observed.

The Feeding Reflex.—In cases where the voluntary movements of the lips and mouth are lost or impaired by bilateral upper motor neuron lesions the approach of food, especially a tasty morsel, towards the mouth may lead to separation of the lips and opening of the mouth, and if food is placed in the mouth, to reflex chewing.

An allied reflex excited by contact is often demonstrable in infants and in stuporose states; touching or stroking the lips causes smacking and chewing movements.

CHAPTER XI

The Visual System

RAYS of light entering the eye cross in the crystalline lens, pass through the vitreous and, having penetrated the retina, excite impulses in the rods and cones which lie on its outer surface. These impulses are transferred through intercalated neurons to the ganglion cells, the axons of which form the innermost layer of the retina. These converge towards the optic disc where, bending to approximately a right angle, they enter the optic nerve through the lamina cribrosa.

Within the optic nerve the fibres are arranged according to their sites of origin: those from the upper part of the retina lie in the upper part of the nerve, those from the lower in its lower segment. The macular fibres at first occupy the outer sector of the nerve, but gradually move towards its centre in which they run till the chiasma is reached. Each optic nerve carries all retinal impulses from the corresponding eye; those from each point of the retina pass through a definite part of its cross-section.

At the chiasma the fibres from the inner or nasal half of each retina separate from the rest, and inter-digitating in small bundles with those from the nasal part of the other eye cross the middle line and join uncrossed fibres from the temporal half of the opposite retina to form the optic tract. The decussating fibres do not, however, cross directly into the optic tract, but after passing the mid-line curve forwards a short distance into the proximal portion of the opposite optic nerve, which consequently contains here, in addition to fibres from the ipsilateral retina, others from the nasal side of the opposite eye (Fig. 24).

Owing to the partial decussation of the optic nerves, the middle or centre of the chiasma consists of fibres carrying impulses from the nasal half of each retina, which is excited by rays of light from the temporal part of each visual field, while the lateral portions of the chiasma contain fibres from the temporal sides of the retinæ, which convey impulses from the nasal portions of the fields of vision.

Within the chiasma the fibres are arranged in the same manner as in the proximal portions of the optic nerves; the macular fibres lie centrally, those from the upper portions of the retinæ dorsally, and those from their lower quadrants in its ventral or basal part.

The anatomical relations of the chiasma to the base of the skull are of considerable clinical importance; the most important variation is the lengths of the intracranial portions of the optic nerves. When these are short the chiasma lies directly above the sella turcica, when long some distance behind it (Fig. 25). Disturbances in the fields of vision caused by a tumour of the pituitary body may consequently vary according to the position of the chiasma in relation to the sella.

Each optic tract contains fibres from the homonymous sides of the two retinæ, the left tract, for instance, those from the left or temporal side of the left eye, and from the left or nasal side of the right eye, and the impulses they convey are excited by rays of light from the right halves of the visual

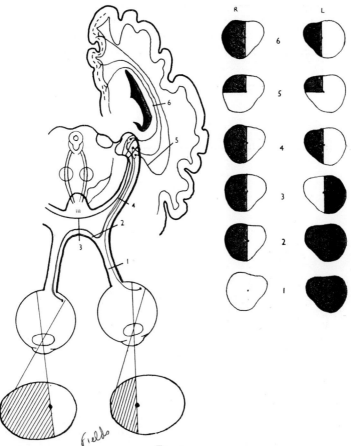

FIG. 24.

Diagram of the course of the visual path from the retina to the occipital lobe. On the right the loss of vision produced by lesions of different levels of the visual system is shown.

fields. Fibres from the maculæ lie in the dorsolateral segment of the tract, those from the upper parts of the retinæ in its dorsal part, and fibres from the lower quadrants of the retinæ in its ventral surface.

The optic tracts pass backwards and upwards round the lateral surface of the mid-brain till they reach the lateral geniculate bodies in which most of their fibres terminate, in fact all except a few which run around the median geniculate bodies to the tectum of the mid-brain; some of these end in the grey matter of the anterior quadrigeminal bodies, others in the pretectal region. These are not concerned in vision, but carry impulses which excite the pupillary reflexes to light falling on the retinæ. A few fibres also end in the pulvinar, but they have probably no visual function. All the fibres of the optic tracts concerned in visual perception terminate in the lateral geniculate bodies.

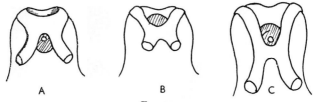

FIG. 25.

The relations of the chiasma to the pituitary when the optic nerves are short *A*—when of average length, *B*—when unusually long, *C* (after de Scheinwitz).

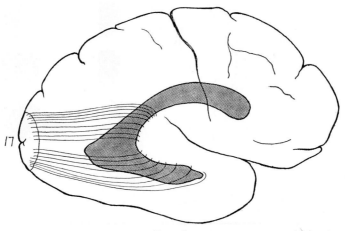

FIG. 26.

Diagram of the optic radiations as its fibres enter the parieto-temporal lobes after curving round the lateral ventricle. Those carrying impulses from the upper and lower quadrants of the retinæ are shown as separate bundles (after Cushing).

The macular fibres end in synapses in the dorsal part of the lateral geniculate ganglion, those from the upper portions of the retinæ in its medial part, and fibres from the lower quadrants enter its lateral segment. Those coming from corresponding points of the two retinæ terminate in close proximity, though probably not around the same cells: there is evidence that they may end in alternate layers of the same region. There is, therefore, a close correspondence, perhaps a point-to-point representation, of corresponding parts of the two retinæ in the lateral geniculate bodies, but it is doubtful if fusion of impulses from their corresponding points occurs at this level.

The optic radiations, or geniculo-striate bundles, which are the final link in the visual system, take origin in the lateral geniculate bodies, and carry visual impulses to the occipital cortex, where they end in the striate area around the calcarine fissure. They take a tortuous course on their way to the occipital lobe (Fig. 24). At first they run lateralwards through the retrolenticular segment of the internal capsule, where they may be involved together with the motor and sensory projection tracts, and then around the lateral ventricle to the white matter of the parieto-occipital lobe, where they form a broad band chiefly in the external sagittal layer. In the latter they turn backwards towards the calcarine cortex. The radiations extend further forwards than is often recognised; part of them, especially the lower fibres, enter the temporal lobe and reach its anterior third before bending in a loop backwards to the lower part of the sagittal laminæ (Fig. 26).

Within the radiations, too, there is a topographical arrangement of fibres according to the source of the retinal impulses they carry: those from the upper quadrants of the retinæ pass along its upper or most dorsal portion, those from the lower parts of the retinæ in the lower or ventral segment of the radiations. The frequency with which a clear-cut quadrantic loss of vision results from partial lesions of the radiations indicates that fibres carrying impulses from the upper and from the lower quadrants of the retinæ respectively are anatomically separate. The position in the radiations of fibres conveying impulses of macular origin is undetermined: they probably run in the lateral portion of its middle segment, but do not form a compact bundle.

The cortex concerned in visual perception is distinguished by a line of medullated fibres, Gennari's line, parallel to its surface, and is consequently known as the striate area. It covers the walls of the posterior calcarine fissure and the adjacent mesial surface of the hemisphere, but it also extends to the occipital pole, and often for a short distance over its lateral surface.

Different areas of the retinæ are represented separately in the visual cortex, the upper quadrants in its upper portion, the lower in its lower, the macular regions in its most posterior part near the occipital pole, and the peripheral segments in its most anterior part which extends slightly beyond the parieto-occipital fissure (Fig. 27).

This projection of each half of the retina on the visual cortex of the opposite hemisphere is spatially exact in the sense that in it are reproduced the relative positions of retinal points; in fact, if one striate area is flattened out it presents a map of the opposite halves of the retinæ, its posterior portion corresponding to the macular region, its anterior part to the periphery of the retina, the floor of the calcarine fissure to the horizontal radius, and portions above and below the latter to the upper and lower retinal quadrants. As rays of light entering the eye cross in the lens, the topographical representation of the visual fields is reversed, their lower quadrants being projected on to the upper portion of the visual cortex and their upper on to its lower (Fig. 27).

In such a map it is evident that the extent of representation of different portions of the retina varies greatly, that of macular or central vision being relatively much larger than that of peripheral vision; as in the motor cortex, the more highly specialised functions are most extensively represented.

Both clinical and physiological investigations show that each point of the retina is linked exclusively to a definite area of the striate area. This rigid localisation explains the constancy and permanence of defects of vision due to lesions of the visual cortex and of the optic radiations.

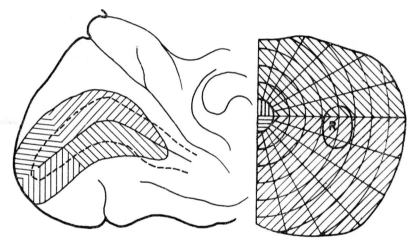

FIG. 27.

To show the representation of the right half of a visual field in the left striate area. The lips of the calcarine fissure, which has been opened up, are represented by a broken line.

Owing to the systematic arrangement of fibres carrying impulses from different portions of the retinæ, and consequently serving determined parts of the visual fields, it is as a rule easy to determine exactly the sites of lesions involving the visual system.

Division of one optic nerve produces complete blindness of this eye, but if the lesion is incomplete those portions of the field served by the injured fibres only suffer. Owing to the greater vulnerability of macular fibres to many processes affecting the transverse section of the nerve, and especially to diffuse disease, central vision is liable to suffer first and most severely; inflammatory lesions, compression and stretching of the nerve, tend to produce central scotomata with intact or less disturbed peripheral vision. Central scotomata may also result from the action of poisons to which either the macular elements or the afferent fibres from them, are susceptible.

When the nerve is injured in the immediate neighbourhood of the chiasma the decussating fibres from the nasal retina of the opposite eye may be also involved, and loss of vision in the opposite temporal field is then associated with blindness or amblyopia of the ipsilateral eye (Fig. 24).

Affections of the chiasma cause more complex disturbances of vision. Lesions of its centre, which interrupt the decussating fibres carrying impressions from the nasal halves of the two retinæ, cause loss of vision in the temporal parts of the fields, or bitemporal hemianopia. Nasal hemianopia of the eye of the same side results from injury of the lateral part of the chiasma. Frequently, however, one optic nerve or one tract is involved at the same time causing either a larger loss of vision on the same side, or a contralateral homonymous hemianopia, in addition to the effects of the chiasmal lesion.

Lesions of the retro-chiasmal portions of the visual system, that is, of the optic tracts, lateral geniculate bodies, optic radiations and calcarine cortex, produce homonymous disturbances of vision which may extend over the whole half of each field or be limited to some portion of it. The loss is usually congruous, that is, identical in size and position in the right and left eyes, but when the radiations are involved it is occasionally incongruous and is then usually greater in the opposite eye in which the temporal field is lost.

In hemianopia due to supra-geniculate lesions the blindness frequently does not extend up to the fixation point; there is a so-called "macular escape" which may extend from 2 to 5 degrees. In this area, however, vision is rarely intact; acuity, and especially colour perception, is often reduced. It has been attributed to bilateral projection to the cortex of macular or central vision, to bifurcation in the chiasma of fibres carrying macular impressions, and to other anatomical arrangements of which there is, however, no evidence. It can be explained by escape of part of the extensive macular area in the cortex, or of some of the fibres conveying macular impulses, which are probably widely distributed in the radiations. This explanation is consistent with the fact that central vision alone may persist when both occipital lobes are injured. Macular escape is, however, often more apparent than real. It may be due to defective or fluctuating fixation of the eye, or to voluntary deviation of it in the patient's efforts to see as far as possible towards the blind side. One explanation which has been put forward is that as a result of blindness of half the fields of vision there is a functional rearrangement in the retina, and the area of most distinct vision is displaced towards the seeing side; a false macula, or "pseudofovea," is developed.

Injuries of retrochiasmal portions of the visual system never cause isolated loss of colour vision; when the perception of colour is impaired

perception of light is always affected too, though often to a less pronounced degree. Patients suffering with so-called pure word blindness,
which is generally a result of a lesion on the under surface of the left
temporo-occipital lobe may, however, be unable to identify colour though
visual acuity is undiminished. This is, however, a form of colour agnosia
rather than loss of colour vision.

Patients are frequently unaware of loss of vision due to suprageniculate
lesions, and consequently may not refer to it in describing their symptoms;
for in contrast to infrageniculate lesions there is rarely subjective dimness
or darkness in the blind portions of the fields.

Examination of Vision

This should begin with estimation of central vision for both near and
distant objects. Snellen's letters and Jaeger's types are usually employed
for this purpose. It is, of course, essential that errors of refraction are
corrected, and that account is taken of the state of the media and of the
retinæ.

Each eye should be tested separately while the other is occluded by a
light bandage or other suitable means.

The peripheral limits of the fields should then be mapped out by
moving a test object slowly and at a uniform rate from beyond the limit
of normal vision towards the point at which the patient's eyes are directed.
It must be borne in mind that a moving object is the most effective
stimulus to the peripheral portions of the retina; a stationary object may
not be seen here, or perceived only when attention is focused on it.

The normal field extends laterally beyond 90 degrees from the fixation point, but its nasal side conforms with the size and shape of the
nose. The upper margin of the field may be restricted by a drooping lid
or an overhanging brow; the lid should then be raised and the head tilted
backwards.

The remaining portions of the field are then examined by exposing a
small object against a uniform or contrasting background at various
angles from the fixation point. By this means large areas can be explored
rapidly. If a scotoma exists its size and shape should be estimated by moving the test object from the blind or amblyopic area towards the normal
parts of the field. Tests should be first carried out by a white object of
medium size: discs 5 to 10 mms. in diameter are usually employed, but
smaller and larger test objects should be available as by means of them
the degree of loss and its position in the field can be observed and
recorded. Perception depends not only on the size of the test object, but
also on its distance from the eye; it is the visual angle subtended by the
object which determines the potency of the stimulus.

Observations made by the use of white objects can be confirmed by
using coloured discs; red and green are the colours most frequently

employed for this purpose. They are particularly useful if the loss of vision is incomplete, as slight disturbances are more easily demonstrated by coloured than by white objects. It must be remembered that the colour fields are much smaller and more dependent on the size of the test object than the fields to white. Coloured test objects may also reveal defects due to retinal lesions in areas in which perception of form and white are little affected.

The field of vision can be investigated either by a perimeter, or by moving the test object by hand against a suitable background. In the latter method, which is known as *confrontation*, fixation is obtained by making the patient look directly at one of the observer's eyes. Though it does not furnish accurately measurable observations such as can be obtained by the perimeter, confrontation possesses many advantages; fixation can be controlled, which is often difficult in inattentive patients, and a larger number of tests can be made before the subject tires. It is often the only method possible in bedridden or helpless patients. A little experience makes it possible to determine approximately the size and position in the field of any defect of vision which may be present, and by varying the size of the test object the degree of disturbance can be estimated.

As in even normal persons the field becomes smaller and the replies less accurate as the subject tires, it is advisable to interrupt the examination for a time, or rest the subject, if there is any sign that his attention is flagging.

By the use of a perimeter the limits of the fields and the state of vision within them can be recorded. A self-recording instrument can be employed, but a simple arc of at least 90 degrees on which the angles of deviation from the fixation point are marked is in many ways preferable.

The perimeter is often regarded as an instrument of precision, but the results obtained by its use depend on many conditions. In the first place, it is less easy to detect deviation of the patient's eye from the fixation point; in the second place, the mechanical movement of the test object frequently produces a sound which attracts the subject's attention and causes him to look towards it, or to reply before it is visible. The results also depend to some extent on the rate and regularity of the movement, which are less easy to control than in confrontation. Consequently the details of the fields recorded by one observer are comparable only with those obtained under identical conditions.

The central portions of the fields can be more minutely examined by any form of a Bjerrum's screen at a distance of one or two meters from the patient, but it cannot be usefully employed for visual angles greater than 30 degrees. In neurological, as opposed to ocular disease defects of the peripheral visual fields can usually be satisfactorily demonstrated on the screen.

The results obtained by all these methods of examination depend to some extent on the degree of illumination, the contrast of the background and the test object, the saturation of the latter if it is coloured, and its rate of movement, as well as on its size. The size of the object and its distance from the eye should always be recorded: this is preferable to stating the visual angle subtended by it—a 3 mm. disc at 300 mm. from the eye subtends about 0·5 degrees. By a useful convention 3/330 indicates the object employed was 3 mm. in diameter and 330 mm. from the eye.

Attention Hemianopia.—When a subject's attention is poor, or when it tires, his replies to stimuli, especially to those falling on the periphery or less sensitive portions of the retinæ, tend to be inaccurate and unreliable. Under these conditions the visual fields, particularly when mapped out by a perimeter, become gradually smaller and their contours irregular. This is frequently so in hysteria and in states of exhaustion.

A specific local loss of visual attention in the hemiopic halves of the visual fields, or in some portion of them, may, however, result from cerebral lesions involving the opposite parieto-occipital lobe. When it is present the field may be normal and isolated stimuli perceived with accuracy, but no response may be obtained, or only a proportion of the stimuli are perceived, on the affected side when attention is diverted or claimed by another stimulus. This can be demonstrated by the observer holding up his two hands, one on each side of the fixation point and at approximately equal angles from it, and requesting the patient to reply to every movement of a finger or thumb. Regular responses are obtained if a finger on either side only is moved, but on simultaneous movements of the fingers to both the right and left, that on the affected side is not perceived or a proportion of them only may be noticed. The intensity of the stimulus to the affected side has little influence on this phenomenon; it may, for instance, be demonstrated by using a test object 1 cm. in diameter on the normal side and one of 20 cms. on the other.

When vision is reduced in the homonymous halves of the fields the responses to small objects may be irregular and inconstant; it is therefore necessary to exclude visual defects and to use large stimuli in testing for visual inattention.

OPHTHALMOSCOPIC EXAMINATION

The ophthalmoscope is an essential instrument for every physician, and particularly for every neurologist, as it reveals changes in the retina due to general and local disease, the state of the retinal arteries which belong to the same system as those of the brain, and the condition of the nerve fibres which carry retinal impulses to the central nervous system. It is in these fibres where they are collected into the papilla or optic disc that the neurologist is chiefly interested.

Ophthalmoscopic examination should be systematic, and a convenient method is to observe in the following order, the outlines of the disc, its colour, the presence or absence of swelling, the state of the normal central cup, and the size and state of the arteries and veins both on the surface of the disc and in the retina. Finally, the retina should be explored, and especially the macular region, but as a rule this cannot be done easily unless the pupil has been dilated by a mydriatic.

VISUAL DISORIENTATION

It is largely by vision that we acquire knowledge of space and recognise the position of objects in it. Localisation in space is not, however, a simple perception nor an innate faculty; it is acquired in childhood by correlating and integrating other sense impressions with visual perceptions. It depends, therefore, on the integrity of anatomical paths by which visual perceptions can be linked with muscular and tactile impressions from all parts of the body, including the ocular musculature, and probably on other sensory afferents too. These are the physiological basis of the psychical judgments on which spatial localisation depends.

The more prominent disturbances of visual orientation result from bilateral lesions of the parieto-occipital regions of the brain, and especially from those which involve the subcortical white matter in the neighbourhood of the angular gyri, but defective localisation in homonymous halves of the visual fields may be caused by injury of this portion of the opposite hemisphere.

Relative localisation, or the ability to recognise the relative positions in space of two objects to one another, may be distinguished from absolute localisation or the recognition of the spatial relation of a visible object to self, though both are generally affected together. Localisation in the coronal plane depends mainly on the local signs of the retinal points excited by the image of the object. The estimation of distance is a more complicated process which requires integrations of impressions of various origins, as those provided by binocular vision, proprioceptive impulses from the ocular muscles, especially those excited by convergence and accommodation, and judgments based on distinctness, light intensity and the comparative size of familiar objects. Stereoscopic vision, which is related to the estimation of distance, may be affected at the same time.

As a result of visual disorientation a patient may be unable to find his way about even in familiar surroundings, and, owing to the failure to recognise the positions and distances of objects, he may collide with obstacles, and may even walk into a wall though he sees it distinctly. He is also unable to grasp or point accurately to objects within the range of his vision.

Topographical memory is often disturbed too; the patient is then unable to visualise or describe routes with which he is familiar, as how to go from one room to another of his house, or from his home to a neighbouring shop or station. Occasionally the distinction of right and left of his own body or of space is lost: this may complicate acts in which visual guidance is required.

Visual memory, or ability to visualise familiar persons and objects, may be also defective.

Disturbances in visual orientation can be readily detected, but it is first essential to exclude defects in the visual fields which may interfere with perception necessary for the tests. The patient should be, in the first place, asked to touch or point in the direction of any object within his range of vision and to estimate its distance from him by sight alone. Relative localisation is tested by describing the relative positions in space of two objects: when it is defective he is unable to count correctly dots on a sheet of paper or coins scattered on a table, and he usually fails to divide a line accurately or to find the centre of a circle. If able to walk he should be required to find his way about a room in which various obstacles, as chairs and tables, are placed, or through a house, and to describe a route with which he is familiar. On attempting to read he often fails to follow the lines, and especially to bring his eyes to the left of the succeeding line.

Unilateral loss of orientation produces less obvious symptoms and is usually not recognised by the subject, but he is unable to point to, or otherwise indicate, the position of an object in the affected homonymous halves of the fields of vision.

CHAPTER XII

Movements of the Eyes

EACH eye is moved by six muscles, two of which, the external and internal recti, deviate it respectively outwards and inwards in the horizontal plane. The other muscles have more complex actions but for practical purposes the superior and inferior recti respectively elevate and depress the eyeball when it is in the abducted position. The superior oblique depresses and the inferior oblique elevates the adducted eye. All the muscles acting in the vertical plane also exert less important activity in rotating the eyeball (Fig. 28).

RIGHT EYE   LEFT EYE.

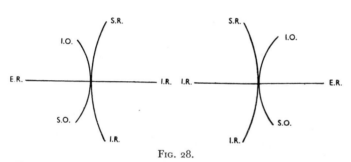

FIG. 28.

Diagram of the direction in which the different external ocular muscles
move the eyes.

The external rectus is innervated by the sixth or abducent nerve, the superior oblique by the fourth or trochlear. These nerves arise from small nuclei in the pons and mid-brain respectively, and each supplies one muscle only. The third, or oculomotor, nerve supplies the remaining four external muscles as well as the levator of the upper lid and the internal musculature of the eye. Its nucleus, which is situated in the central grey matter of the upper part of the mid-brain ventral to the aqueduct of Sylvius, consists of a series of more or less well-defined groups of cells each of which is generally assumed to supply efferent fibres to a single muscle. There are divergencies of opinion on the exact localisation of function within the nucleus and opportunities for anatomical veri-fication are rare. Clinical observations, however, indicate that the fibres to the pupil take origin from its most anterior part, probably from the collection of cells known as the Edinger-Westphal nucleus. From im-mediately behind this the fibres to the elevators of the globes spring. The next group of cells probably innervates the internal rectus, while

III

the inferior rectus probably receives fibres from the posterior extremity of the nucleus which extends towards the trochlear nucleus in which the nerve to the superior oblique, the other depressor, takes origin (Fig. 29). This is the order in which ocular movements are affected by lesions extending caudalwards from the oral portion of the mid-brain.

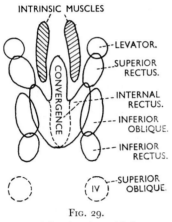

FIG. 29.

The origin in the third nerve nucleus of the fibres to the separate ocular muscles (Brouwer).

For accurate vision it is necessary that the images of the object on which the eyes are directed should fall on corresponding parts of the two retinæ. This is, under normal conditions, determined by the conjugate action of those muscles which deviate the eyes in each direction and the relaxation of their antagonists. On looking to the right, for example, the right external rectus and the left internal rectus contract synchronously and to an equal degree so that the visual axes remain parallel when a distant object is in vision.

The co-ordination of the muscles which contract in any movement of the two eyes depends on subcortical mechanisms, that concerned in vertical movements and convergence being in or near the superior colliculi, but the existence of a pontine centre for lateral deviation has never been substantiated. Most, if not all of the symptoms thought to arise from a lesion of this hypothetical centre could equally result from a lesion of the medial longitudinal bundle connecting the sixth and third nerve nuclei. Supranuclear lesions involving these conjugate mechanisms, or fibres carrying impulses to them, consequently cause palsies of movement of both eyes in a definite direction, not paralysis of muscles. This may be seen in a case of paralysis of lateral movement to one side, as the eye which fails to turn inwards when this movement is attempted adducts normally on convergence; though the internal rectus is paralysed in one movement it contracts normally in the other (Fig. 30).

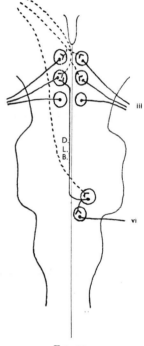

FIG. 30.

Diagram of the probable connections of the oculomotor nuclei. The supranuclear paths are represented by broken lines. D.L.B., the dorsal longitudinal bundle.

In the cortex of each hemisphere of the forebrain there are areas which when stimulated in both lower animals and in man excite movements of the eyes. That in the second frontal gyrus is probably concerned with voluntary deviations: on electrical stimulation of it movement of both eyes to the opposite side is generally obtained, but vertical movements can also be elicited. The projection fibres from this frontal centre run to the brain-stem with pyramidal fibres.

Ocular movements can also be obtained from the cortex within or around the visual or striate area in the occipital lobe: these are concerned with visual reflexes (p. 98). Fibres from this region pass directly to the mid-brain and pons. Ocular movements elicited by stimulation of the temporal lobes probably represent reflex deviations induced by the perception of sounds by the auditory centre.

Ocular Palsies

Ocular palsies are among the most common neurological symptoms. One or more muscles may be paralysed, and it is often important to determine which is involved. This is usually easy when one muscle only is affected and the weakness is of considerable degree, but often difficult when the paresis is slight or more than one muscle is weak. If the rules by which paresis of a single muscle can be recognised are understood multiple muscle palsies can be worked out.

One of the most prominent symptoms is *squint or strabismus*, the affected eye being deviated in the direction opposite to that in which the weak muscle should move it, for example, inwards when the external rectus is paralysed. But squint may not be visible when the weakness is slight.

Secondary deviation of the normal eye in the direction of action of the weak muscle occurs when a screen is placed in front of it and the patient fixes an object with the affected eye; it is sometimes more obvious than the squint.

The head may also be tilted in the direction of action of the weak muscle in order that the latter may not be called upon to contract on looking at an object. When the right external rectus is feeble the head may be rotated to the right, but head tilting is generally more prominent when an oblique is involved; if, for instance, the right superior oblique is paretic it is bent forwards and the chin turned to the right.

Erroneous projection, which also occurs in the direction in which the weak muscle normally moves the eye, can be demonstrated by covering the normal eye and asking the patient to point to an object on which the affected eye is fixed. The error increases as the object is moved in the direction of action of the weak muscle.

Diplopia, or double vision, is the most distressing and constant symptom of an ocular palsy. It is due to failure of the images of the object towards which the eyes are directed to fall on corresponding parts of the two

I

retinæ; the images are consequently projected separately into space, and the patient perceives them separately.

When an ocular paresis is slight double vision may be present though there is no obvious squint or defect in movement, or there may be no conscious doubling of the object, but merely blurring or indistinctness of its outline. Diplopia can then, however, be generally demonstrated by placing differently coloured glasses in front of his eyes as the patient looks at a light. When an ocular palsy is of long duration, the patient may learn to suppress the false image and thus get rid of diplopia.

It is by a study of the relative positions of the projected images that the muscle or muscles at fault can be most accurately determined. This can

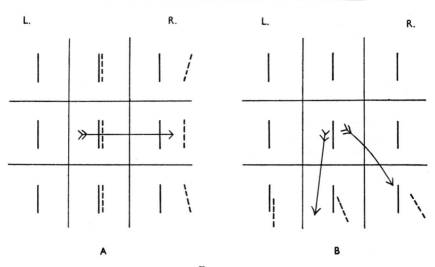

Fig. 31.

Diagrams of the relative positions of the true and false images in cases of palsy of the right external rectus, A, and of the right superior oblique, B.
The firm lines indicate the positions of the images of the normal eye, the broken lines those of the paretic eye. The arrows show the directions in which deviation of the eyes increases separation of the images.

be carried out by making the patient describe or indicate the relative positions of the two images of a pencil or other linear object held at least thirty inches in front of him. The pencil should be vertical when the separation of the images is mainly lateral, and horizontal when the image is above the other. The image which belongs to each eye can be determined by observing which disappears when one eye is covered.

Diplopia can be, however, more easily studied in a dark room by placing a coloured glass in front of one eye and requiring the patient to describe the relative positions of the coloured and uncoloured images of a candle or linear source of light placed in various positions in his field of vision. In these tests the head should be fixed or held immobile. The observations can be recorded for further analysis on a simple chart on which the relative positions of the two images when the eyes are central and when deviated in the horizontal, vertical and oblique planes are indicated (Fig. 31).

By the following rules the muscle which is weak can be recognised:

(1) The false image is usually less distinct.

(2) Diplopia occurs in those positions of the eyes which depend on contraction of the weak muscle or muscles.

(3) The false image is projected in the direction of action of the weak muscle. This is due to the fact that rays of light which enter the squinting eye from the object on which the normal eye is fixed, form an image on the retina on that side of the macula opposite to the direction in which the weak muscle should move it.

Consequently, a feeble adductor, which causes a divergent squint, produces a crossed diplopia; a weak abductor a convergent squint, but uncrossed double vision.

When a levator is affected the false image lies higher, when a depressor is weak it lies lower than that of the normal eye.

When a rotator is weak the false image is oblique and tilted in the direction of the rotating action of the muscle.

(4) The separation of the images increases when the test object is moved in the direction of action of the weak muscle.

Contractures or shortening of the unopposed antagonists may complicate the picture of diplopia, or the patient may learn to suppress the false image, particularly if visual acuity of the paretic eye is subnormal and the ocular palsy is of long standing.

Squint due to palsy of an ocular muscle must be distinguished from concomitant strabismus, which is commonly divergent. Here the range of movement of the squinting eye is unrestricted, the degree of squint is constant in all directions of gaze and there is no diplopia. Vision is usually defective in the squinting eye.

Conjugate ocular palsies are characterised by abolition or weakness of movement of both eyes in one or more directions. As the muscles that contract together in conjugate movement are equally feeble, there is no squint or diplopia unless, as often happens, an ocular nucleus or nerve is also injured.

The most common conjugate palsy is that of lateral horizontal movement: this results from a lesion on the same side of the pons in the neighbourhood of the nucleus of the sixth nerve. Upward or downward movement may be abolished by disease of the upper part of the mid-brain. Conjugate convergence may also be affected by mid-brain lesions.

In this type of conjugate palsy the eyes fail to move in one or more directions in response to all stimuli.

Supranuclear Ocular Palsies—"Pseudo-ophthalmoplegia."—This results from injury of the projection fibres which carry voluntary impulses to the oculomotor nuclei or oculogyric centres (Fig. 30). The patient is unable to move his eyes voluntarily in one or more directions, but they deviate in response to visual and other stimuli, as a flash of light, or a moving object, a pin-prick, an unexpected sound, and in response to vestibular stimulation. They may also follow an object when it moves slowly, and remain fixed on a point when his head is rotated or tilted. These deviations depend on the fixation reflex which keeps the eyes fixed on the point on which they are directed. When the power of voluntary movement is lost this reflex may become so dominant that the patient has difficulty in disengaging his eyes from an object within central vision. These disturbances are, however, pronounced only in the presence of bilateral disease which, when progressive, may eventually cause paralysis of reflexly induced as well as voluntary movement.

NYSTAGMUS

Nystagmus consists of involuntary oscillating or rhythmic movements of the eyes. It may be due either to visual defects or to disturbances in the nervous mechanism concerned in the movements and postures of the eyes.

Even in normal fixation the eyes are not motionless, but constantly oscillate through small angles so that the images of the object on which they are directed move over the maculæ in order to avoid fatigue of the receptive elements. These oscillations, however, are so fine and rapid that they cannot be recognised by the naked eye.

Nystagmus of visual origin is usually pendular or oscillatory on central fixation; the eyes swing to and fro horizontally or vertically, but there is often a rotatory element too. When the eyes are moved from the ordinary position of rest it generally assumes the form of alternate rapid and slow jerks in the line of deviation. It is commonly associated with amblyopia present from early life, owing to opacities in the media, disease of the maculæ, or gross errors of refraction. It also occurs in association with albinism. Accurate fixation is acquired only some months after birth, but if vision is defective it may never develop, and the eyes then swing round the object at which the child gazes. It occurs also as a congential abnormality in the absence of marked disturbance of vision. Nystagmus may also be associated with head-nodding in children, but in some of these cases at least it seems to be compensatory to movements of the head.

Occupational nystagmus, particularly that which occurs in coal-miners, is also of visual origin but is now rare. It occurred in men working in poor illumination, as in miners on badly lit coal faces. In dark adaptation the peripheral portions of the retinæ are more sensitive than the macular regions and they are therefore employed in preference to central fixation. In order to avoid fatigue no one extramacular point is made use of, but the images of the object at which the miner gazes are switched from point to point on the retinæ by movement of the eyes. These movements eventually become established, even in good illumination, and produce apparent motion of objects seen, which is one of the symptoms of the condition. The oscillations are rapid, generally rythmic, and either lateral or rotatory. They usually increase on deviation of the eyes, especially in upward deviation.

Rhythmic nystagmus occurs in normal persons when the eyes are directed in succession on a series of moving objects, as when a traveller by train looks at the landscape, or when a person watches figures or lines on a rotating drum. The eyes follow one object till it passes out of vision and then spring back to the position of rest till another point again draws them with it. It consists of a slow phase by which the eyes follow the moving object, and a quick phase which corresponds with their return. This so-called optokinetic nystagmus depends on the integrity of paths connecting the occipital with the fronto-central cortex, and is abolished to the opposite side when these are interrupted. In clinical examination it can be tested by the use of a rotating drum on which lines are marked.

Irregular jerks of the eyes are often visible when they are fully deviated, especially in the horizontal plane, but they are rarely so regular as to be confused with nystagmus. They usually cease when the deviation is maintained for a time. Similar irregular jerks of the eyes may be due to irregular or intermittent contraction of weak ocular muscles; they occur only when a weak muscle is thrown into action and when the affected eye is used in fixation. The nature of these nystagmoid jerks can be recognised by covering each eye in succession, as they occur only when the patient fixes with the paretic eye.

Nystagmus can also be evoked by stimulation and by destructive lesions of the labyrinth, but it persists for, at the most, only two minutes after stimulation has ceased, and disappears within a few days of a labyrinthine injury. The jerks occur in the direction of movement of the endolymph, and may be consequently either horizontal, vertical, or rotatory according to the canal or the combination of canals stimulated. It consists of slow deviations of the eyes, usually towards the resting position, and rapid jerks in the opposite direction. The oscillations increase in amplitude on deviation of the eyes in the direction of the quick phase. The slow phase is the essential element, but nystagmus is generally described by the direction of the rapid jerk (see Vestibular System, p. 130).

The only affections of the central nervous system which produce nystagmus are those which involve the central end-stations of the vestibular nerves or their immediate connections. It occurs, therefore, with disease of the pons, mid-brain and cerebellum; it is seen in its most characteristic form in acute lesions of the latter. It is essentially a rhythmic nystagmus, and is usually visible only on deviation of the eyes from their position of rest. It is always more pronounced, *i.e.*, the amplitude of the jerks is greater, on movement of the eyes in the direction of the quick phase, and increases the further the eyes deviate in this direction. In cerebellar disease it is more marked, the jerks being slower and of larger amplitude, on deviation of the eyes towards the side of the lesion but this is less constant in chronic lesions (Fig. 32).

The nystagmus which accompanies cerebellar and pontine disease requires accurate fixation to show its full development, while that which results from irritation or destruction of a labyrinth is usually more pronounced when fixation is made impossible by screening the eyes or placing in front of them high convex lenses. The position of the head may also influence nystagmus, especially that due to vestibular lesions; consequently it should be looked for both when the head is erect and the patient lies supine. Nystagmus due to certain peripheral lesions of the vestibular apparatus may occur only on rapid change of posture and, when the history is suggestive, this point should be specifically examined.

To investigate nystagmus the eyes should first be inspected in their central position of rest, and then when deviated fully to each side, and upwards and downwards. The point on which gaze is directed should be at least twenty inches distant, as hypermetropic eyes may fail to focus and fix it accurately within this distance. It is also necessary to note the character of the movements, their rate and amplitude in different positions, and the positions of the eyes in which they occur. A rotary element is often difficult to detect; it can be most easily seen by watching the displacement of a conjunctival vessel.

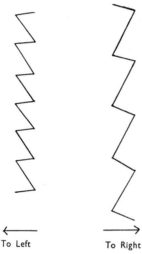

To Left   To Right

FIG. 32.

Diagram of nystagmus in a patient with a lesion of the right side of the cerebellum. On looking to the right the jerks are slower but of larger amplitude than on deviation of the eyes to the left. Read downwards.

PUPILS

The muscle fibres of the iris are unstriated and are innervated by the autonomic system. The circular fibres, which constrict the pupil, are supplied by parasympathetic fibres through the third cranial nerve, the radial dilator fibres by the cervical sympathetic.

The constrictor nerves take origin in the anterior part of the third nerve nucleus, probably from that group of cells known as the Edinger-Westphal nucleus. They enter the trunk of the third nerve, and, passing through its branch to the inferior oblique muscle, terminate in the ciliary ganglion. Here post-ganglionic fibres, known as the short ciliary nerves, take origin, penetrate the sclera of the eyeball and running forward between it and the choroid end in the iris and the ciliary muscle (Fig. 34).

The pupillary fibres of the third nerve are activated by impulses excited reflexly by light falling on the retinæ. These pass along the optic nerves, the chiasma and the optic tract in company with the fibres carrying visual impressions, but when they reach the mid-brain they separate from these and turn around the mesial side of the mesial geniculate body to the pretectal region, and possibly to the roof of the mid-brain, where they end in synapses around cells from which another relay of fibres spring: the latter run to the nuclei of the third nerves (Fig. 33). As each eye sends impulses to both sides of the mid-brain, and as some of the fibres connecting this with the oculomotor nuclei decussate, retinal impulses from each eye reach both nuclei. Consequently, rays of light entering one eye excite contraction of the pupil of that eye, the direct reaction, and also that of the opposite eye, the consensual reaction.

If one optic nerve is divided the pupils fail to respond to light entering this eye, but contract on illumination of the opposite eye, the direct reflex is lost, the consensual reflex is preserved. When an optic nerve is less severely damaged, as by a retrobulbar neuritis, the pupil may contract on direct illumination, but fail to maintain steady contraction though the eye remains exposed to light.

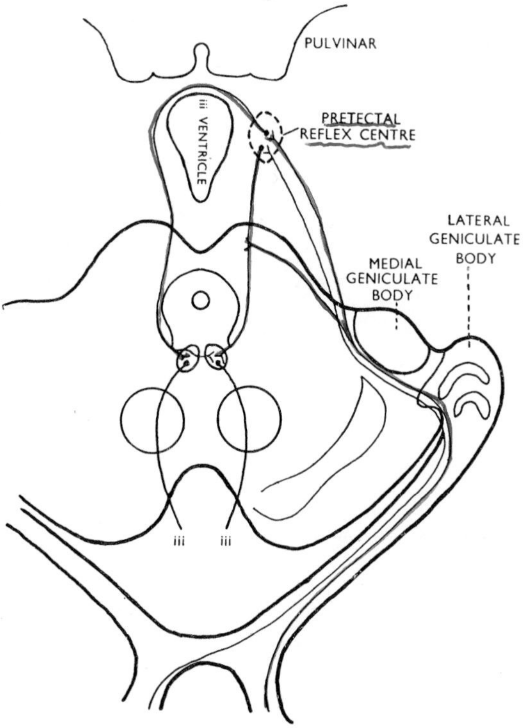

FIG. 33.

Diagram of the probable course of the reflex paths for the response of the pupils to light.

Since the reflex impulses run as far as the lateral geniculate bodies in the same paths as those which subserve vision, blindness in any part of the field of vision owing to an infra-geniculate lesion produces loss of the pupillary response to light falling on the corresponding part of the retina; a left-sided homonymous hemianopia due to a lesion of the right optic tract, for instance, is accompanied by absence of the reflex to light entering the eyes from the left halves of the visual fields. Disease of the visual system above the lateral geniculate bodies does not disturb the pupillary reactions to light.

Any injury of the constrictor centre or of its efferent path in the third nerve, in the ciliary ganglion or in the short ciliary nerves, disturbs the reaction of the pupil to light. The pupil also dilates unless the dilator fibres in the cervical sympathetic are at the same time involved.

The sympathetic innervation is carried by pre-ganglionic fibres of the cervical sympathetic which take origin in the upper two thoracic segments of the spinal cord, and pass up the neck in the sympathetic chain of the superior cervical ganglion where they end; post-ganglionic fibres from this ganglion enter the skull in the sheath of the carotid artery, and after passing through the wall of the cavernous sinus join the ophthalmic

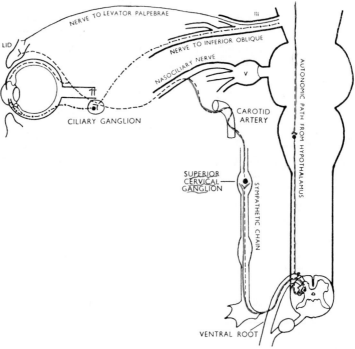

Fig. 34.

Diagram of the course of the oculo-sympathetic fibres.

division of the trigeminal nerve and reach the iris by way of the long ciliary and the nasociliary nerves (Fig. 34). The activity of the oculo-sympathetic system is controlled by the hypothalamus, with which its spinal centre is connected by fibres which pass through the reticular substance of the brain-stem and the lateral column of the cord. Injury of these fibres may produce symptoms similar to those of a cervical sympathetic palsy, but they are usually less pronounced and more transient.

Stimulation of one cervical sympathetic dilates the pupil on the same side, but the effects of negative or destructive lesions are more commonly seen. Then the pupil becomes smaller, but its reflex activity to light remains unimpaired. Dilatation, which can usually be elicited by painful stimuli, as pinching or vigorously rubbing the skin on the same side of the neck, is unobtainable when the post-ganglionic fibres are divided.

The pupils also contract on convergence of the eyes and on accommodation on a near object. This is an associated or synkinetic phenomenon which helps to cut out unnecessary peripheral vision and increase the depth of focus. Convergence is more potent in bringing about contraction than is accommodation. This reaction is abolished by any lesion of the constrictor centre in the oculomotor nucleus or its efferent fibres, or of the ciliary ganglion or the short ciliary nerves, but its main value in clinical medicine is that its presence shows that the pupil is capable of contracting and that movements of the iris are not restricted by adhesions or synechiæ.

The pupils also contract on looking upwards and on vigorous closure of the lids: this may be seen if the closure is opposed by the observer's fingers. This also is a synkinetic reaction.

The response of the iris to various drugs may be used to test the state of its nervous supply. Atropine and homatropine dilate the pupil by paralysing the parasympathetic nerve endings, and eserine and pilocarpine constrict it by stimulating them: these reactions are absent when the ciliary ganglion or the short ciliary nerves are degenerated. Cocaine dilates the pupil by stimulating the sympathetic nerve endings in the iris; it fails to do so when the post-ganglionic fibres are injured.

Under normal conditions the pupils vary in size owing to the relative activity of sympathetic and parasympathetic innervation of the iris, although the influence of the latter is probably by far the more important. Injury of the third nerve and stimulation of the cervical sympathetic dilate them; while certain drugs, as morphia, and paralysis of the sympathetic contract them. The pupils also contract in sleep, but dilate in certain forms of coma. Pain and emotional excitement enlarge the pupils by exciting secretion of adrenaline which stimulates the sympathetic fibres. The degree of illumination of the retinæ is, however, the chief factor in determining their size.

The pupils are, as a rule, equal in size and their outlines are circular and regular. Pronounced inequality may be due to disease of the iris, but is often a result of disorder of its innervation. A progressive widening of the pupils, at first on one side, is a valuable sign of acutely increasing intracranial pressure and is probably due to compression of the oculomotor nerve against the meninges.

Irregularity of outline is frequently the result of local disease, as adhesions or fibrosis following an attack of iritis, but may accompany loss of the reflex to light, especially if this is due to damage of the efferent fibres of the reflex arc.

An important sign in clinical neurology is failure of one or both pupils to react to light though convergence brings about normal contraction;

it consists, therefore, in an isolated loss of the light reflex. Despite the fact that light produces no contraction of the pupil, they are usually abnormally small and their outlines are often irregular. This is a common feature of syphilitic diseases of the nervous system, and particularly of tabes dorsalis and general paralysis. It was first described by Argyll Robertson and is generally known by his name. When it has persisted for a time the iris may become thin and atrophic, and when combined with a certain amount of ptosis produces that expression so characteristic of tabes to the experienced observer. The Argyll Robertson pupil does not dilate readily when atropine is instilled into the conjunctival sac, but stimulation of the cervical sympathetic usually widens that on the same side.

There is considerable doubt as to the site and nature of the lesion which causes the Argyll Robertson phenomenon, but it has certainly occurred with traumatic lesions restricted to the contents of the orbit and is then presumably due to damage to peripheral structures. A similar loss of the light reflex with retention of constriction on convergence has, however, also been described in lesions of the upper mid-brain. When the third nerve or its nucleus is involved contraction on convergence also disappears.

Total ophthalmoplegia interna, in which the pupil fails to contract to light and on convergence, and accommodation is also paralysed, results from disease or injury involving the third nucleus, its nerve, the ciliary ganglion or the short ciliary nerves.

A relatively rare condition, known as the tonic pupil, is characterised by very slow contraction on convergence, and even slower relaxation. The reflex to light is often lost too. One or both eyes may be affected. Its pathology is uncertain, but it is a harmless condition mostly affecting young women.

The reaction of the pupils to light may be tested while the patient faces a window by alternately screening and exposing in succession each eye to illumination, but the reflex may be more easily observed by exposure to a bright light, as that of an electric torch, in a darkened room. The hemianopic reaction is theoretically of value in distinguishing a hemianopia due to disease of the supra-geniculate section of the visual path from that due to a lesion of the optic tract, but it requires the use of parallel rays of light and is not easily demonstrated under clinical conditions.

LIDS

The postures of the lids depend on the relative degree of contraction in the orbiculares palpebrarum which close them, and of the levators of the upper lids and the unstriated muscle fibres within them, both of which hold the upper lids up. Weakness of either group of muscles consequently produces abnormalities of posture.

Each orbicularis is innervated by the facial nerve, and the palpebral fissure consequently becomes widened, owing to slight elevation of the upper and drooping of the lower lid, when a facial palsy is present.

The levator palpebræ is supplied by the oculomotor nerve, and the unstriated muscle the lid contains by fibres of the cervical sympathetic which, on their way to it, pass through the sphenopalatine ganglion (Fig. 34). Ptosis, or drooping of the upper lid, may result from palsy of either of these nerves. If the levator is paralysed the eye cannot be opened at all and paresis causes more or less severe ptosis, partially overcome by contraction of the frontalis. Ptosis due to palsy of the cervical sympathetic disappears on upward deviation of the eyes as contraction of the levator is unimpaired, and is probably responsible for the partial ptosis in tabes.

Less frequently a palpebral fissure is narrowed by excessive contraction of the orbicularis; an intermittent spasm, which may close the eye, is frequently part of a facial spasm. It occurs particularly on bringing other muscles of the face into action, as in showing the teeth or retracting the angle of the mouth.

Lid retraction is a well known sign of thyrotoxicosis but cannot with certainty be attributed to overactivity of the sympathetic supply. A somewhat similar retraction of the upper lid occasionally accompanies ocular palsies in which the levator is not involved, and occurs particularly when upward movement of the eyes is defective. In the latter case it is probably a synkinetic phenomenon accompanying vigorous attempts to look upwards, with which rising of the upper lid is normally associated.

The lids are occasionally involved in other abnormal associated movements, the best known of which is jaw-winking. Here there is usually a permanent ptosis which is frequently congenital, but the upper lid rises, sometimes excessively, on opening the mouth or on chewing.

CHAPTER XIII

Special senses; Smell, Taste and Hearing

THE olfactory receptor organs in the nasal mucosa are selectively sensitive to minute concentrations of molecules in the air in the naso-pharynx. The sensation aroused is variously interpreted as a smell if the stimulus is derived from the environment or as a taste if derived from food or drink. All tastes except those of salt, sweet, acid and bitter depend on the integrity of the olfactory system.

In man the sense of smell has little function except in adding to the enjoyment of life and providing an occasional warning of fire or gas. Traces of its overwhelming importance in many lower animals survive in its extraordinary power of the vivid evocation of long-buried memories. This is no doubt a relic of evolutionary times when the memories evoked were not those of some childhood scene but of vital distinctions between food or poison, friend or foe. The primitive and atavistic nature of the sense of smell is reflected in its central nervous connections. From the olfactory bulb on the inferior surface of the frontal lobe neuronal chains reach a wide area of cerebral cortex, without passing through the thalamus. Although many comparatively primitive structures in the forebrain have been included in the rhinencephalon it is probable that in man only a small area of cortex in the region of the uncus of the temporal lobe is directly concerned with the appreciation of smell.

A complaint of loss of sense of smell, not due to nasal obstruction, implies damage to the receptor organs or their immediate central connections on both sides as unilateral loss passes unnoticed. Refined testing can demonstrate relative and asymmetrical reduction in olfactory acuity and discrimination in a great variety of lesions of the cerebral hemisphere but these changes are of no practical importance.

Sense of smell may be tested crudely by holding aromatic substances below each nostril in turn with the other blocked and asking the patient, with his eyes closed, to state if he smells anything. Bilateral loss is easily detected but the spread of air inspired through one nostril throughout the nasal cavity is so rapid that unilateral anosmia may be difficult to distinguish with certainty. A false claim to have lost the sense of smell may sometimes be detected by using ammonia which irritates the somatic endings in the nasal mucosa, supplied by the trigeminal nerve, and not the olfactory organs. Inability to detect ammonia is therefore nearly always hysterical. Patients should not be asked to identify smells by name as this is a peculiarly difficult task, the answers being greatly influenced by the environment. The most homely kitchen smells if used in a test in hospital are usually identified as some noxious medicament.

Positive symptoms also occur. With incomplete peripheral lesions taste and smell may be unpleasantly distorted and may persist in the absence of the stimulus. A smell, unpleasant and indescribable, but instantly recognisable to the patient, is a classical form of aura in temporal lobe epilepsy.

Taste. The afferent pathways from the taste buds of the tongue and palate are remarkably complex. From the posterior third of the tongue impulses are conveyed in the ninth cranial nerve but, although this area is the most sensitive, no simple means of testing it in isolation can be devised.

Fibres from the anterior two-thirds run in the lingual nerve but then join the chorda tympani to pass through the ear and join the facial nerve. The ganglion cells are in the geniculate ganglion. All gustatory afferents eventually concentrate in the tractus solitarius in the medulla but the more central connections are conjectural.

The sense of taste is most commonly affected in lesions of the facial nerve and may be an early or even an isolated sign. The traditional method of examination consists in placing small quantities of powder or concentrated solutions of salt, sugar, quinine or citric acid on one side of the protruded tongue and asking the patient to point to what he considers the correct taste written on a card. This is a time consuming, inaccurate and uninformative method, partly because that part of the tongue that can be reached is not plentifully supplied with taste buds. A much simpler method is to apply the terminals of a torch battery to each side of the tongue in turn and ask if the current can be felt. The "taste" of a battery does, in fact, reach consciousness through the gustatory fibres and not through the trigeminal fibres of common sensation.

Hearing. The auditory receptor organ is the organ of Corti in the cochlea. In the great majority of those complaining of either negative or positive symptoms the defect lies in the middle or inner ear, preventing the normal access of sound waves to the receptor organ or injuring the receptor itself. Many disease processes of the inner ear may also damage the cochlear nerve so that mixed forms of deafness are common. Lesions of the cochlear nerve without peripheral damage are important but far less common.

The central connections of the impulses concerned with hearing are scarcely less complex than those of the visual system. A similar precise localisation of function both in the intermediate cell station, the medial geniculate body, and in the superior gyrus of the temporal lobe, also probably exists but is of little clinical importance as there appears to be complete bilateral projection. Unilateral deafness from central lesions is not, therefore, encountered and there have been only occasional reports of bilateral deafness due to symmetrical lesions beneath the temporal cortex. The clinical problem is nearly always that of distinguishing deafness due to peripheral causes from that due to a lesion of the cochlear nerve.

For most clinical purposes it is sufficient to test hearing by blocking one side with intermittent pressure over the tragus and speaking in an increasingly loud voice until the patient can repeat what is said. High tones can be tested with a ticking watch or by the noise made by rubbing the fingers together. The traditional tuning fork tests are usually admirable in confirming deafness obviously due to middle ear disease but in most other circumstances are unreliable. A high pitched tuning fork (512) is struck and placed on the mastoid process. When it is no longer audible it is held to the meatus. In the normal or in moderate degrees of nerve deafness the note will still be heard but in middle ear disease it will not. Mixed types of deafness cannot usefully be investigated in this way.

The *audiogram* can be used to distinguish between disease of the receptor organ and of the cochlear nerve. In the former the percentage loss of hearing decreases as the stimulus becomes louder; the phenomenon of recruitment. This does not occur in a cochlear nerve lesion where the percentage loss remains approximately the same throughout the range of retained hearing.

The common positive symptom affecting the acoustic system is *tinnitus*. This again is nearly always due to peripheral disease and is often an intractable symptom. Anxious patients become aware of the normal sound of the pulse when lying on one ear in bed. A complaint of arterial bruits audible to the examiner occurs with sufficient frequency to warrant the use of the stethoscope in every case of tinnitus.

Auditory hallucinations occur in temporal lobe epilepsy but are nearly always highly organised and not simple notes or sounds. A tune, a duet or even a full orchestra and chorus may be heard but the melody can never be remembered afterwards. In contrast to olfactory hallucinations the sensations are nearly always pleasant or even ecstatic.

CHAPTER XIV

Postural Reactions and the Vestibular System

THE importance of the muscle spindle and the stretch reflex in movement and the maintenance of posture and the control of these spinal mechanisms by higher nervous centres was discussed in Chapter V. The regulation of posture is so complicated and so deeply below the level of consciousness that it cannot be properly studied in intact persons, and only rarely and incompletely in disease in man. Its functions have, however, been partly unravelled by experiments on animals which isolated its components for separate study: these experiments revealed how important and intricate a part it plays in the determination of posture and preservation of equilibrium. Many of the conclusions which have been drawn from these experiments are certainly applicable to man, but it is a striking fact that these activities seem less essential here, though the biped gait and erect posture over a narrow base must require a more efficient mechanism for the reflex control and maintenance of equilibrium than suffices for quadripeds. The afferent impulses which activate them come particularly from the muscles of the neck and trunk, from the labyrinths and probably from the eyes, though in man visual reflexes require the intervention of the cerebral cortex.

Neck Reflexes.—Dorsiflexion of the head of a decerebrate animal leads to extension of the fore-limbs and flexion of the hind-limbs, so that the posture assumed is that of looking up. Forward flexion of the head produces the opposite reaction; the animal lowers the forepart of its body and extends its hind-limbs as if inspecting the ground below its snout. Rotation of the head to one side leads to extension of the fore-limb of the side towards which the chin is moved and flexion of the opposite limb. These reactions depend on impulses from the muscles of the neck; they occur when afferents from all other sources are cut out.

Neck reflexes are less easy to demonstrate in man, but when the motor centres of the forebrain are damaged, or when a deeper unilateral lesion causes a hemiplegia, rotation of the head to the paralysed side may extend the ipsilateral arm and flex the opposite limbs (Fig. 35). These reflexes may modify or influence other reactions. If, while his head is straight, a hemiplegic patient clenches his normal hand vigorously there is usually flexion and adduction of the paralysed arm, but if his head is turned to the hemiplegic side flexion may be replaced by extension of the limb. On the other hand, flexion and adduction of the arm are increased by rotation of the head to the unaffected side. The tendency of the inexperienced driver of a motor-car to deviate from the direct line on turning his head suddenly is probably due to reflexes from the muscles of his neck, which are not yet under purposeful control.

The Labyrinths.—The postural mechanisms of the mid-brain are, however, mainly activated and controlled by impulses conducted by the vestibular nerves from the labyrinths, which are also proprioceptive organs. These impulses excite extensive muscular contractions necessary for the maintenance of equilibrium both at rest and during movement. Owing to their structure the labyrinths are affected by the position of the head in space and by its movements in all directions.

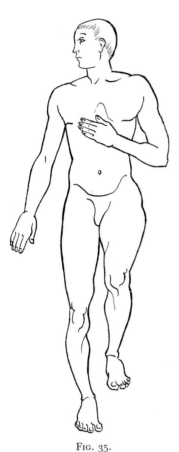

FIG. 35.

In a case of right hemiplegia passive rotation of the head to the right may cause extension of the right and flexion of the left limbs.

Each labyrinth consists of two parts: three semi-circular canals, which are arranged at right angles to one another and consequently correspond to the three planes of space; and two cavities, the utricle, into which the semi-circular canals open, and the saccule.

Within the bony canals there are membranous canals of similar shape which contain fluid—endolymph. One end of each canal is dilated into an ampulla, and each ampulla receives on its sentient surface a branch of the vestibular nerve, which is stimulated by flow of the endolymph when the head moves in its plane. Movement of the head in any direction may consequently excite labyrinthine impulses, but angular acceleration is probably the most effective stimulus.

The utricle and saccule also receive fibres from the vestibular nerves; these enter them only at special points, which are known as the maculæ. When the head is erect the macula of the utricle is horizontal, that of the saccule vertical. Fine hair-like processes of cells which serve as receptors extend from each macula into a gelatinous substance on its surface in which small calcareous granules, known as otoliths, are embedded. The weight or draw of these otoliths on the receptive hairs naturally varies with the position of the head, and therefore signals its position. While the semi-circular canals react to movement, the otolithic organs are in position to respond to postures, and are consequently static organs, but there is evidence they also react to linear acceleration. The utricle is certainly such an organ, but it is doubtful if the saccule has this function, though as its macula is at right angles to that of the utricle, they would together form an efficient organ from which postural responses could be excited.

In animal experiments destruction of the vestibular nuclei abolishes decerebrate rigidity but in man lesions of the vestibular system cannot be shown to exert any influence on the tone of the limbs.

Impulses conveyed centralwards by the vestibular nerves enter the caudal portion of the pons and are widely distributed, either directly or indirectly, to the brain-stem and cerebellum. The highest centre for labyrinthine reflexes seems to be within the mid-brain at the level of the red nuclei. There is evidence that this centre is connected with the cortex of the temporal lobes of the fore-brain.

Though impulses of labyrinthine origin do not under normal conditions reach consciousness, labyrinthine disturbances produce definite symptoms which are, however, usually intermittent. The mildest of these, which is usually termed "dizziness" by the patient, is merely a sensation of unsteadiness or lack of balance, often accompanied by a feeling of movement within the head, without, however, apparent motion of either the patient himself or of the outer world. Dizziness, however, is not always of labyrinthine origin or a result of labyrinthine disease but has a multitude of causes. It is often due to circulatory disturbances, as a sudden fall of blood pressure, as in syncope, or in diminished blood supply to the head on suddenly rising from the horizontal position. It may also accompany hypertension. In some of these cases it is more probable that dizziness is due to disturbance of circulation in some portion of the central nervous system rather than to disorder of function in the labyrinth. The term is used by patients to describe almost any unfamiliar sensation in the head.

The term "vertigo," on the other hand, should be reserved for attacks, usually of short duration, in which there is sensation of movement of the environment and/or of the patient himself, with disturbances of equilibrium. It may be accompanied by other symptoms due to spread of impulses of vestibular origin through the brain-stem, as nausea, vomiting, palpitations, slowing of the pulse, disorders of vision and often sweating or sensations of heat or cold.

These, which are the essential subjective features of acute labyrinthine disorder, are usually accompanied by objective signs, the chief of which are disturbances of balance, involuntary displacements of the limbs and trunk, deviation of the eyes and nystagmus. The nature of the pathological changes to which they may be due vary but consist essentially of asymmetrical loss or diminution of vestibular function.

This characteristic form of vertigo is usually of labyrinthine origin: the fact that it is often associated with loss or diminution of hearing in one ear at least, and with tinnitus or with changes in the excitability of the vestibular organs points to this origin, but transient attacks, often limited to apparent movement of objects or of self, may result from functional or structural disturbances in its central nervous connections.

K

When one labyrinth is suddenly destroyed the patient, if erect, inclines to that side, his trunk and head rotate in the opposite direction, and, if his arms are extended in front of him, they deviate to the opposite side. This deviation of the arms is the basis of so-called *past-pointing*; a normal person can, when his eyes are closed, bring a finger with approximate accuracy to a point he had previously seen, but after destruction of one labyrinth his finger deviates towards the affected side. This test is best performed by making the patient extend the limb fully and place his index finger in contact with an object, as the observer's finger, then lower or raise his arm and attempt to bring his finger to it again. If the point to be touched is the middle of a scale held horizontally the amount of each deviation can be measured. Conclusions should not be based on a single test, for when there is pathological deviation the error in direction usually increases on repeated attempts. A similar test can be carried out for movements in the horizontal plane, and can be applied to the lower as well as to the upper limb.

The most constant symptoms on destruction of one labyrinth are however, deviation of the eyes and *nystagmus* with its quick phase to the opposite side, due to the unbalanced activity of the normal labyrinth. In man they are transient and generally disappear after a few days, althought they may reappear briefly on movement of the head.

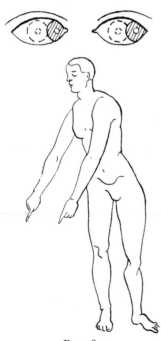

The functional activity of the labyrinths may be tested by inducing currents in the endolymph of the semi-circular canals either by rotation of the head or by thermal stimuli. Each canal can be stimulated by tilting the head so that it lies in the plane of rotation, but this method has the disadvantage that the canal of the other side which is in the same plane is also excited. Rotation away from the ampulla is, however, more effective than towards it; rotation to the right when the head is erect, for instance, affects chiefly the left horizontal canal.

Rotation Test.—This test can best be carried out by seating the patient on a revolving chair with his head supported by a suitable rest, and fixed so that the canal to be tested lies in the plane of rotation; he is then rotated ten times at a uniform rate in about twenty seconds. During rotation the endolymph at first tends to lag behind the movement of the head, but when rotation is suddenly arrested it continues for a moment, owing

Fig. 36.
The reactions to irrigation of the right ear with cold water.

to its inertia, to move in this direction. If during rotation the endolymph current was towards the ampulla, when rotation ceases it is for a moment away from it. Consequently, the stimulus and the reactions it evokes during and after rotation are corresponding opposites.

As the reactions which occur during rotation cannot easily be observed, attention is devoted to those which appear when it is arrested. When the patient is placed on his feet he inclines and tends to fall in the direction of rotation and his arms deviate in the same direction, especially in movement: this becomes apparent in tests for past-pointing. The nystagmus which follows rotation is, however, the most important indication of the functional state of the labyrinth; it consists of rapid jerks of the eyes in the opposite direction to that of rotation and slower deviations in the direction of rotation. It becomes more obvious when the patient looks about 45 degrees in the direction of the slow phase and increases when accurate fixation is cut out by placing convex lenses in front of his eyes, or by other means. The intensity of the reaction can be measured by the duration of the nystagmus; it generally lasts about half a minute.

The *Caloric Test* is carried out by running either cold or warm water into the external meatus of one ear. It can be standardised by always using water of the same temperatures, as 30° C. and 44° C., that is, approximately the same number of degrees below and above the temperature of the body, and by continuous irrigation through a nozzle of standard calibre for forty seconds. Unfortunately, only the external canal can be tested by this method, as being nearer the meatus it is most affected by alterations of temperature. The reactions are greater when this canal is vertical; this position is obtained when the patient lies on his back and his head is tilted forward to about 30 degrees; cold water then induces a flow of endolymph from the ampulla, warm water towards it; the effects are therefore complimentary.

The results obtained by this test are similar to those elicited by rotation. Irrigation of the right ear with cold water is followed by a tendency to fall to the right, past-pointing in the same direction and horizontal nystagmus with its quick phase to the left (Fig. 36). When warm water is employed the reactions are in the opposite directions. The excitability of the canal can be measured by the duration of the nystagmus, the average being about two minutes.

Unilateral or bilateral *canal paresis* is shown by reduction or failure of response to both hot and cold water on one or both sides, asymmetrical loss being detected more reliably. In most contexts this can be taken as evidence of disease of the peripheral portion of the vestibular nerve.

A lesion of the central vestibular connections may produce *directional preponderance*. Here the duration of the nystagmus to the side opposite to the lesion is reduced, that is to say the response to cold water in one ear and to hot in the other. This sign is often difficult to interpret and the caloric test itself requires scrupulous attention to detail.

CHAPTER XV

Epilepsy and Loss of Consciousness

THE clinical problem of unconsciousness is sharply divided between the patient in coma and the patient, apparently perfectly well, complaining of a single or of repeated attacks of loss of consciousness.

The difficulties encountered in explaining any form of transient coma may be illustrated by that common cause, head injury resulting in concussion. The mechanism by which a blow on the head can render a patient unconscious without any apparent permanent ill-effects is not fully understood. The concept of widespread or universal dysfunction of the neurons of the cerebral cortex resulting directly from the injury has little to recommend it. The reticular formation in the brain-stem is currently held to exert, directly or indirectly, an alerting effect on the entire cerebral cortex. If this is indeed included in the numerous functions of this comparatively small neuronal complex, a temporary disturbance at such a central site would be a rational explanation for sudden loss of consciousness. A similar mechanism probably accounts for coma in rapidly enlarging intracranial lesions such as a tumour or haematoma as, if the patient dies, the brain-stem is usually found to be severely distorted or the site of haemorrhage.

Many external toxins and internal metabolic disorders cause coma but remarkably little is known of the effects of such agents at cellular level or even of their site of action in the brain. Unconsciousness in meningitis, encephalitis or subarachnoid haemorrhage without evidence of focal brain damage is similarly accepted without further thought as a symptom natural to such diseases, but its immediate cause remains obscure.

The underlying causes of recurrent attacks of unconsciousness are much less numerous but much more difficult to diagnose. Even the most detailed history may be fruitless as the patient may know little or nothing of his symptoms. Whenever possible an eye-witness should be questioned.

Neuronal function depends on a continuous supply of oxygen and glucose and failure of either causes unconsciousness. Spontaneous hypoglycaemia of this degree is uncommon and usually causes prolonged confusion and amnesia rather than sudden coma. Cerebral anoxia is common and occurs in fainting from any cause, from Stokes-Adams attacks and in transient cerebral ischaemia secondary to atherosclerosis. Syncope is usually easily recognised by the circumstances of the attack; the sudden rising from a chair, a hot crowded room, a painful injury or minor trauma. Heart block can be detected clinically or by the electrocardiograph. The diagnosis of transient cerebral ischaemic attacks from vascular insufficiency is more difficult and to some extent depends on the exclusion of other causes and the obvious presence of atherosclerosis.

By far the commonest important cause of attacks of loss of consciousness is *epilepsy*. It is naturally impossible to deal with this vast subject in detail and only certain aspects of what is known of its causation and clinical manifestations can be discussed. Some over-simplification is unavoidable.

Idiopathic epilepsy forms a distinctive clinical entity of which the essential feature appears to be that the abnormal electrical discharge responsible for the fits begins in central structures. The precise site of origin has not been determined but the result is immediate generalised dysfunction of the cerebral cortex (Fig. 37a).

In the *major fit* both negative and positive symptoms occur. The patient falls unconscious and has a generalised convulsion. Most attacks start with momentary tonic spasm of the whole musculature, which is generally uniform, but if greater on one side may rotate the head and deviate the eyes, or involve more intensely one arm or leg. The upper limbs are usually flexed, the lower are more commonly extended, the head is retracted, the jaws are clenched and the face is grotesquely distorted. Spasm of the chest may cause a cry or groan, and the arrest of respiration leads to congestion. The attitudes produced by tonic spasms are entirely purposeless and unnatural.

Within a few seconds the tonic spasms relax and give place to intermittent clonic convulsions, by which the whole body is more or less simultaneously involved, but their severity may vary in its different parts. They last on an average about one minute, but irregular isolated jerks may continue for several seconds. When the tonic spasm of the thorax subsides air enters the lungs and the patient regains his colour. Frothy saliva is often extruded between the lips; it may be blood-stained if the tongue or lips were caught between the teeth while the jaws were in clonic spasm. Incontinence of urine is common; it may be evacuated in jets during the clonic stage, or may dribble away during the subsequent phase of relaxation.

The dramatic features of a convulsion often divert attention from the post-convulsive stage, but this may provide equally valuable information. For a time there is complete muscular relaxation; if a limb is raised it falls inertly; in falling, the hand may strike the face heavily without exciting any reaction; the deep reflexes are unobtainable and the plantar responses are extensor or abnormal.

Consciousness returns slowly after some minutes, but the patient usually passes into a deep sleep without having regained full contact with his environment. This is an important point in the diagnosis of a generalised epileptic convulsion. On waking memory of events immediately

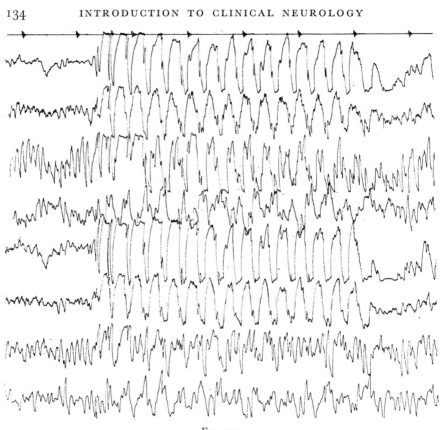

Fig. 37a.

Fig. 37.

Electroencephalographic recordings.

In both tracings the top four lines are recorded from the right side of the head and the bottom four from the left. (*a*) Shows the simultaneous appearance of slow waves and spikes in all areas, indicating that the abnormality originates in central structures. (*b*) Shows a fundamentally different form of epileptic disturbance in that irregular slow waves and spikes are almost continuously present over the left hemisphere, in fact mainly over the temporal lobe.

preceding the seizure is often lost or defective, and for a time the patient may be confused, disorientated, resistive or even violent.

In *petit mal* the negative symptoms predominate. Consciousness is instantaneously lost for a period seldom exceeding a few seconds. The patient does not fall and incontinence of urine is most uncommon. The face may flush or go pale. Positive symptoms are confined to occasional flickering clonic movements of the facial muscles or hands. The end of the attack is equally abrupt and there is no subsequent confusion although the thread of conversation may be lost. Some patients are unaware of having petit mal. Although much less dramatic these attacks share with the major fits of idiopathic epilepsy the immediate loss of consciousness without warning.

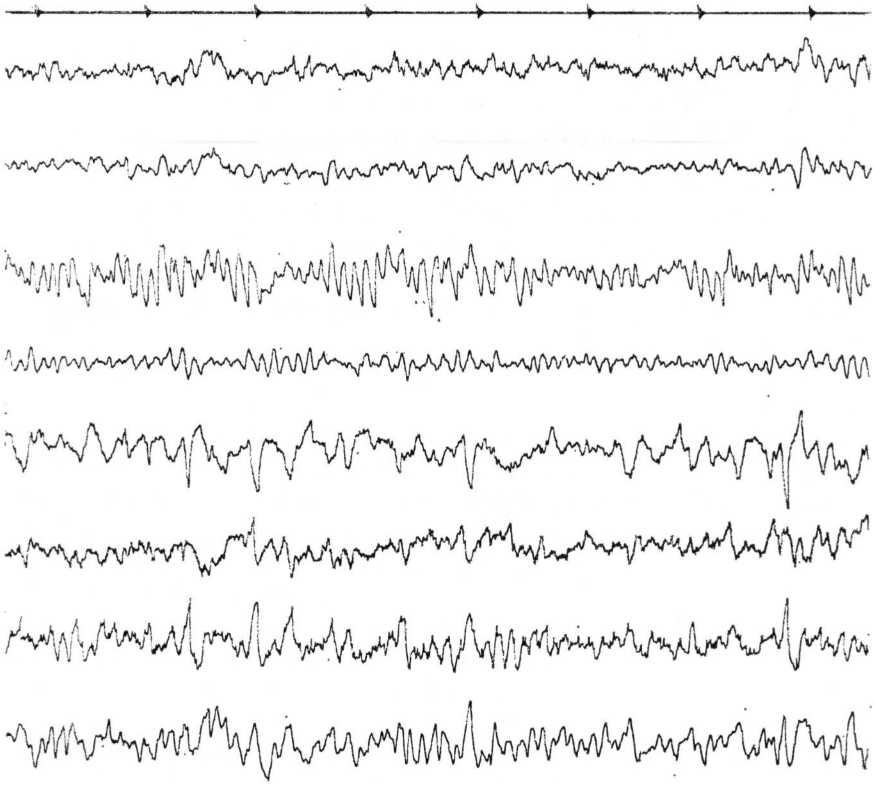

FIG. 37b.

Some patients with idiopathic epilepsy, particularly those with petit mal, also have myoclonic jerks, usually of the arms and nearly always confined to the early morning.

The syndrome therefore consists of the onset of major fits or petit mal or both in childhood or adolescence in patients otherwise perfectly normal. Even here, where the epilepsy is the only sign of disease, it should be regarded as a *symptom* and not as a disease entity. The cause of the centrally situated abnormal activity has not been determined but probably only because the biochemistry of the brain is insufficiently known.

Major fits, without warning, and indistinguishable from those of idiopathic epilepsy may occur in patients with obvious brain disease. In many such patients, however, there is evidence that the abnormal electrical discharge did not begin centrally but originated locally in some specific area of the cerebral cortex (Fig. 37b). This is most obvious in the *focal motor fit* or Jacksonian epilepsy. Here the essential feature is that the convulsion *begins* unilaterally. The commonest sites of origin are those in which movement can most readily be provoked by electrical stimulation of the motor cortex; the thumb and index, the big toe and the angle of the mouth. Clonic jerking spreads in a more or less regular manner to neighbouring structures but it is rare to be able to witness the orderly "march" thought to indicate the spread of the abnormal discharge through the motor cortex.

The anatomical lesions responsible for the occurrence of focal convulsions generally lie in the neighbourhood of the motor cortex and may involve it, but it is essential that they do not damage seriously the functional activity of the cells in which the discharge begins. Local motor discharges are, however, occasionally associated with more distant disease which, it must be assumed, affects the activity or raises the excitability of the discharging point.

As a rule the spasms of local epilepsy are at first clonic owing to intermittent contraction of one set of muscles and reciprocal relaxation of their antagonists, but if the discharge becomes more vigorous all the muscles of the part are involved, the antagonists as well as the agonists pass into tetanic spasm. Frequently, however, an intense discharge evokes from the onset contractions of all the muscles of a part and fixes it in an attitude that is determined by the relative power of the muscles involved. Though this is often described as a tonic phase, when handled the muscles can be felt contracting intermittently or clonically.

Neither the movements produced by an epileptic discharge nor the positions into which they bring a limb have a purposive character or the features of a designed act; the muscular contractions lead only to an irregular and purposeless discord of movement. This is particularly obvious when more specialised motor functions are involved, as phonation or articulation; forcible expulsion of air through a partly closed glottis by contraction of the thorax may produce a cry or groan, but never an articulated word or conventional symbol of expression.

The clonic stage of a local seizure is usually followed by paresis of voluntary movement of the parts which were convulsed; there may even be complete paralysis for several minutes or even for hours after severe attacks. During this period the tone of the muscles and the knee-jerks and other stretch reflexes are depressed, but the plantar response is extensor if the lower limb is involved. This paresis is generally regarded as due to functional exhaustion of the cortical grey matter which was involved in the discharge, but may in fact be evidence of continued abnormal discharge from the affected neurons.

A focal motor fit may stop at any point or may be followed immediately by a major fit. If present theories are correct this must mean that central structures have secondarily been thrown into disorder and that the resulting diffuse discharge has caused diffuse dysfunction.

Focal discharges in areas of cerebral cortex remote from the motor area may similarly cause focal fits or major fits preceded by focal features. It is these various initial symptoms that comprise the *aura* which may therefore be of great localising value.

Focal Sensory Epilepsy.—A discharge which involves the sensory cortex in the parietal lobe, either alone or combined with a motor discharge, excites subjective sensations of various forms. They are generally described by the patient as tingling, numbness or deadness, but even when spoken of as "loss of feeling," they seem to be always positive symptoms. Occasionally the sensation is of movement, a feeling that a portion of the body, usually a segment of a limb, has moved. There is never an illusion of a complicated act.

These sensations are referred to the opposite side of the body, and spread in a manner similar to the march of a motor seizure, or like this they may be limited to a portion of it, most commonly to a hand or foot, or to one side of the face. They may even be referred to a phantom limb. Their march is, however, often less regular than that of a motor attack; they may, for instance, spread directly from a hand to a foot without involving intervening portions of the body.

Sensory attacks are usually followed by transient diminution of sensibility in the parts to which the sensations has been referred. Those forms subserved by the cortex naturally suffer most severely, especially recognition of the position of the limbs in space and identification of objects in contact with them, but even painful stimuli, which are mediated through subcortical centres, may not be felt with normal acuity. This is due to functional depression of these closely related structures; it is analogous to the spinal shock which follows an acute lesion of the motor cortex or of its projection fibres.

Visual Seizures.—Excitation of the occipital cortex may induce visual sensations which are projected to the corresponding portions of the visual fields over which they usually appear to move. These visual sensations are always simple and usually crude, as coloured or uncoloured lights or flashes, or a star or ball. Frequently they are not identified with a definite perception, but described merely as "something there," or "something moving."

Loss or diminution of vision in the portion of the field to which these phenomena had been referred usually follows an attack.

As mentioned above major fits without an aura may occur in patients with proven focal cortical lesions. This may be explained by the absence of any recognisable sensation arising from stimulation of that particular cortical area. Fits very similar to the classical petit mal of idiopathic epilepsy may occur in children undoubtedly suffering from brain damage. This is almost certainly explained by the site of the cerebral damage, which in children anoxic at birth often involves central structures.

Temporal lobe epilepsy—This is far more common than other types of focal fit, possibly because the temporal lobe may be peculiarly vulnerable to minor injury at birth. Here again the pattern is that of the focal fit in isolation or forming the aura or initial stage of a major fit. Many such patients may, in addition, have major fits without warning.

The focal symptoms are remarkably interesting and highly variable. The common aura of an epigastric sensation rising to the head is thought to originate in the temporal lobe. Unpleasant hallucinations of smell or taste are common. Sensations of dreaming with vivid stereotyped visual hallucinations occur but can seldom be described in any detail by the patient. They often seem to resemble an experience of a state of being rather than a disordered function limited to one or more of the special senses. An aura may consist of a psychic experience alone, here again nearly always unpleasant and difficult to describe. Far less well defined symptoms summarised by the patient as "dizziness" are common but true vertigo may also occur.

The behaviour of a patient during an attack of temporal lobe epilepsy is often characteristic of a *psycho-motor fit*. The patient appears confused rather than fully unconscious and carries out co-ordinated but inappropriate movements, quite different from the clonic jerks of a motor fit. Smacking the lips, rubbing the hands together, muttering, fiddling with papers or beginning to undress are among the commonest activities seen. These differ in no respect from the *automatism* that sometimes occurs *after* a major fit and which then also strongly suggests a focal temporal lobe origin.

Many forms of epileptic fit are difficult to classify. For instance attacks involving brief loss of consciousness with a few clonic jerks are common in children and are clearly neither major fits nor petit mal. A category of *minor fits* must be retained but whenever possible a full description of what is actually observed is worth far more than an attempt at rigid classification.

If epilepsy is to be approached in a rational and humane manner it is important to emphasise that an epileptic fit is always a symptom and is not a disease. It may indeed be the only symptom but this is due to our ignorance of the underlying defect in idiopathic epilepsy or to justified reluctance to submit every patient to the full rigours of neurological investigation. The word "epileptiform" can be discarded as it has lost its original meaning of a fit not due to some hypothetical epileptic *disease*.

CHAPTER XVI

Speech and its Disorders

THE term speech, in the sense it is used by neurologists and psychologists, signifies the expression of thoughts by auditory and visual means for their conveyance to others, and the comprehension of the ideas of others by means of their spoken and written words.

This use of spoken and written words to express our thoughts and receive the thoughts of others is known as *external speech*, but it depends on *internal speech*, that is, the formulation in our minds of unuttered words. It includes, in addition to the mental processes that are expressed in external speech, those concerned in the comprehension of speech of others. Our thoughts deal predominantly in terms of speech; words and verbal symbols can be regarded as the coins of mental commerce. It is, for instance, a general experience that during preoccupation not only do we formulate our ideas in words, but may even form or utter words subconsciously.

Speech is consequently a product of mind, a psychological as well as a physiological function, by which mind can be exteriorised for the purpose of communication with our fellows, but it is also an instrument of mind, for without speech our mental activities are restricted. A speechless man is not, however, necessarily thoughtless.

It is impossible here to touch on the many facets of the complicated faculty of speech, or to review even the more important hypotheses which have been put forward to explain the processes on which it depends and their disorders by disease, but a short, though hypothetical, sketch of how man developed the power of speech may facilitate an understanding of the subject.

By means of expressions, attitudes and sounds animals are undoubtedly able to express their emotions at least; for instance, a cry associated with pain, or a sound that repeatedly accompanied the pangs of hunger or other instincts and feelings, comes to signify to its companions the suffering or the desires of the animal that utters them; one cry becomes a symbol of hurt, another a symbol of hunger or desire for food. In apes the use of such symbols to express emotions, desires and even rudimentary thoughts is undoubtedly more highly developed, but in man only has the use of symbols in thinking and in expression of thoughts reached that stage when it can be referred to as speech.

We can picture to ourselves the primitive man who first employed sounds as a vehicle for the expression of thought. He had not advanced far beyond the intellectual level of his ancestors to whom the utterance of a simple sound signified little more than an emotion, but he gradually learned to employ other sounds, at first perhaps applied to concrete objects only, and to recognise their significance when they were uttered by his fellows. Thus "Ma" may have signified mother, and some other elementary sound corresponded to food or desire for nourishment. In this way words, or auditory symbols, came into use. Sounds which became words were, however, and have remained conventional symbols, but each of them has been invested with an arbitrary though definite connotation. As greater and a more highly differentiated power of articulation was acquired they became more numerous and more differentiated. The vocabulary grew gradually, providing more names for concrete objects and for abstract qualities possessed by them. Later there was acquired the use of other sound-symbols, or words, to connect or relate those first acquired to one another, to one's self or to some other object, and modifications of words served to indicate number, time and conceptual relations. In this way sentences were acquired; this extended enormously the utility of speech.

That evolution may have followed some such course is suggested by the method by which the growing child acquires the power of speech. The significance of names, or sounds applied to objects, is first apprehended; then the child learns, after many attempts, to utter and apply the same sounds to these objects. Later, he succeeds in combining words into sentences, and becomes able by the use of verbs to say something about persons and things, by adjectives to qualify or add to the meaning of the word he uses, and to indicate the relations between them by other elements of speech.

Speech is consequently the use of symbols to express thoughts, and at first auditory symbols, or spoken words, only were employed. These word-symbols are, however, only conventional; they vary in different languages, but in each language they become fixed and standardised. The first essential step in the development of language is appreciation of the significance of these conventional symbols. If their significance is not learned, as in congenital deafness, speech is not acquired naturally, and when speech is lost they can no longer serve as a vehicle for thought and its expression; words become only a medley of sounds like those of an unknown foreign tongue.

At a later stage of his development man found it necessary to record his thoughts more permanently than by spoken words, which when uttered are, as the breath which carries them, gone for ever. Drawings or pictures were first employed for this purpose. Later these became less life-like and largely symbolic, as the hieroglyphs of the ancient Egyptians, but they remained merely pictorial representations of objects, not records of their conventional names. Original Chinese script also represented things without the use of words or names; for instance, a drawing of a roof with the figure of a woman beneath it represented a home, but it was merely a pictorial representation or pictograph. Even later, when less concrete ideas were expressed by the use of visual symbols, as when a roof with the figures of two women beneath it came to signify a quarrel, Chinese script was only the symbolic expression of ideas, or ideograms, and was wholly unrelated to the words that express these ideas in speech.

Writing, on the other hand, is the recording of auditory symbols by graphic symbols. A separate symbol might be selected for each word and modification of a word, but this would be a cumbersome and inflexible method. The first stage in the development of writing, as we understand it, was the breaking up or analysis of the complex sounds of words into a number of simple elements, which when rearranged and combined are capable of representing all the sound-symbols or words of the language, and many scripts appear to have passed through a phase of linking the syllabic sound, the phoneme, with a graphic symbol. This has many advantages but is less flexible than the alphabetic system eventually adopted in most civilisations where each symbol corresponds, in theory, to a single consonant or vowel sound. The complexities of spelling have, however, to some extent restored the entire word as the essential symbol rather than its individual letters. In writing and reading, therefore, we employ symbols of symbols, for writing is built up of visual symbols of auditory symbols. Writing and reading are consequently largely dependent on auditory speech, and are more unstable and vulnerable than it in disease. They are also more artificial faculties than articulate speech; they are learned by each individual later in life, and may not be acquired in the absence of education; in fact, many races, some of which possess highly developed languages, as the Cree Indians of North America, have never learned to record their words by visual symbols.

It is, however, propositions, or a series of words in which something is stated, affirmed or denied, not words themselves, which are the units of speech. Single words are meaningless unless related to other words; even "Yes" has a meaning only when it signifies "I will do it," or "I have done it," or "I agree to what you say," or other affirmation.

Speech consequently consists in the formulation of propositions in mind, their expression by spoken or written words, and the comprehension of such propositions when presented by others by sounds or in writing.

The formulation of propositions is a psychological function, and the comprehension of speech when heard or read in print is psychological too, but like all psychological functions they must have a physiological basis. The expression of propositions in spoken words and in writing is, however, a physiological process; the organisation, grading and the co-ordination, as well as the execution, of the movements of the larynx, palate, tongue and lips, and of those of the fingers which guide the pen, are dependent on the integrity of localised anatomical structures.

It is therefore obvious that speech is essentially a mental process by which formulæ or patterns are determined in which our ideas can be communicated to others by means of auditory (words) or visual (writing) symbols, and by which we are enabled to understand the significance or import of such symbols when made use of by others.

Language is not, however, the only mode of expression available to man: gestures and pantomime can serve the same purpose. Gestures are primitive and limited in scope, but by pantomime or dumb-show more complex ideas can be made accessible to others. Both suffer when internal speech is disturbed. Finger language and lip-reading, as practised by deaf mutes, are also forms of speech, and in aphasia suffer equally with articulate expression and its comprehension.

Special tests are necessary to reveal fully the nature of the various disturbances of speech met with in clinical work, but, as in the case of other functions, much can be learned by observing the behaviour of the patient and his reactions in ordinary intercourse. Since all functions of speech are disturbed to some extent by an affection of any constituent of it, it is difficult to classify satisfactorily the many manifestations of aphasia, but for clinical purposes we may distinguish forms in which comprehension is mainly affected from those in which expression of thought by spoken and written words is more seriously involved.

Receptive or Sensory Aphasia.—The essential feature of this form of aphasia is inability to understand the significance of words spoken or written by others. This may amount to complete loss of comprehension, or there may be partial defect only. In complete sensory aphasia the patient is unable to understand and respond correctly to verbal communications, whether spoken or written; no question or order evokes a reply, and the significance of gestures is defective or lost, but drawings and pictures may be recognised, provided they portray the natural appearance of objects. Such an order as "Close your eyes," or "Open your mouth," conveys no idea of what is required, but a response may be obtained if the observer performs the action at the same time as giving the order.

More frequently the lack of comprehension is not complete. Then, as a rule, it is the names of objects or of abstract qualities attached to them which suffer most severely. To the order "Close your eyes" the patient may respond by closing his mouth, or when asked, "Give me the blue pencil," he may pick up one of any colour from a series in front of him. The longer and the more complicated the question or order is, the greater is the difficulty in carrying it out. For instance, he may succeed in placing a coin on a table when told to do so, but fail in any stage of the action when requested to put one coin on the table, another in his pocket and hand a third to the examiner. Similarly, the question, "When did your illness begin?" may evoke a correct reply, but when asked, "How and when did you become ill?" he may fail to reply accurately, though each predicate may be understood separately. The patient is reduced to dealing with simple and isolated verbal communications: simple sentences may be comprehended; compound sentences, that is, those containing two or more predicates, present greater difficulty; while complex sentences, in which in addition to the main clause there are two or more subordinate clauses, are not comprehended.

As letters and printed words are visual symbols of auditory symbols, comprehension of writing and print is always defective too, and when the aphasia is incomplete these functions are often those most severely affected. Even the individual letters may not be recognised; more commonly there is inability to recognise the words they form when properly arranged.

The recall of words for the purpose of expression of thought is closely associated with the physiological mechanisms through which the significance of spoken words is appreciated, and consequently when the comprehension of speech is defective, the patient is usually unable to express himself accurately. If has often been assumed that the recall of words depends on the existence of "verbal images" or "memories of words" which are stored as such in circumscribed areas of the brain. Internal speech on which communication of ideas to others depends is, however, a psychological activity, and such images can be only mental phenomena: they are not concrete or pre-formed, but come into existence only when elaborated in mind from traces or memories of past experiences; then they can serve as patterns or schemes for the motor acts by which speech is expressed. Failure to recall words is therefore not due to destruction of stocks of pre-formed images, but to disorders of the mental processes by which such images are evoked and associated with corresponding ideas.

In severe degrees of sensory aphasia speech is mere jargon, consisting of unconventional or unintelligible sounds, or wrong words may be used, or words may be omitted or wrongly arranged in sentences. As he is unable to comprehend spoken language the patient is usually unaware of his own mistakes and fails to perceive that his jargon means nothing to others; the failure of his hearers to understand him is often attributed to their stupidity.

In less severe degrees words and even simple sentences may be used correctly, but they cannot be combined accurately to express a train of thought. The chief and often apparently the only defect is nominal aphasia or difficulty in recalling names of objects, which are often described by their qualities or use: a knife may be "Something to cut with," a ball, "A round thing." Grammatical structure is often incorrect; words may be omitted or misplaced, or wrong words used, definition or qualification by adjectives and adverbs may be omitted, or intended relations insufficiently described. Though the patient may be able to respond by "Yes" or "No," and even express simple propositions by words, he fails to explain himself in a series of sentences and is consequently unable to take part in ordinary conversation.

Words which cannot be recalled spontaneously may be, however, evoked from without. If asked, "Do you mean a knife?" after he has failed to name the object, he may reply, "Yes, of course it is a knife," and may continue to use the term correctly, or may apply it as a name for other things. This tendency to perseveration, that is, to employ repeatedly a word that has been recently uttered, often regardless of its propriety, is a common feature of this type of aphasia. When asked to name a series of objects the first of which is a knife, he may call all the others "knife." Simple word formulæ, as "I am well," may be the only response to a series of different questions, and even "Yes" or "No" may be used indiscriminately.

As a rule, there is an even greater disorder of writing: well-known words are incorrectly spelled and letters may be omitted or replaced by unrecognisable signs. This inability to write correctly becomes apparent in both spontaneous efforts and in writing to dictation: in the one case, there is a failure to formulate words in visual symbols; in the other, to translate rapidly auditory into visual symbols. If the significance of such simple visual symbols as individual letters is preserved, copying print into cursive script may be possible.

Motor Aphasia.—The term motor aphasia, which has been hallowed by use, can still be employed to signify failure or defect in the expression of internal speech by articulate sounds, but other disorders of speech are usually associated with it.

The enunciation of words requires long series of delicate movements of the larynx, palate, tongue and lips, which must be arranged in accurate sequence. In motor aphasia all these elementary movements may be undisturbed, but they cannot be combined to produce articulate speech; there is an *apraxia* of these acts, an inability to build up complicated acts from series of simple movements. Though paresis of one side of the face and of the tongue may accompany motor aphasia, they are not in any way responsible for it. The inability of many aphasics to protrude their tongues to order, though they can do so under other conditions, as in licking their lips, is a common instance of apraxia (p. 155).

Motor aphasia is therefore characterised by inability to combine and integrate those movements by which audible speech is produced though the individual movements are unimpaired. Internal speech may remain intact, a defect in the formulation of propositions is not its cause; it is due to inability to reproduce the requisite patterns of movement of verbal expression. In severe degrees no word may be possible, but the patient may occasionally utter, usually under emotional stress, single words or phrases, often expletives or "Yes" or "No," which, however, cannot be regarded as elements of speech, as they are usually inappropriate or do not represent propositions, and may not express his thoughts. In less severe disorders, or as recovery takes place, simple words or phrases may be employed either correctly or wrong in part, for instance, "I want breaker" for "I want breakfast"; simple patterns of movement are available, but not the more complicated patterns which underlie longer words.

Perseveration is common; when a word or short phrase has been success-fully uttered the patient may continue to use it in reply to subsequent questions. In milder degrees the most prominent features are slow and stumbling utterance, hesitation in finding words, the use of wrong or mutilated words, hesitancy and lack of the normal rhythm which fre-quently supplements spoken language in the expression of thoughts and emotions.

A similar, but usually a more severe degree of agraphia, or inability to express speech in writing, generally accompanies motor aphasia; it is, in fact, doubtful if a patient with aphasia can ever express himself as well with the pen as in articulate speech. This is an important point in the distinction of motor aphasia from anarthria and hysterical mutism, in which expression of propositions in writing is not affected.

Pure motor aphasia is rare; comprehension of speech is generally involved to a minor degree at least, and the use of numbers is often disturbed.

Localisation of the functions of speech has been the subject of much controversy. On the one side anatomical diagrams have been propounded in which representation of its separate elements are confined to narrowly circumscribed areas of the cortex; and, on the other side, it has been argued that as speech, in so far as it is the formulation of propositions in verbal symbols, is a mental process it cannot be a function of small isolated por-tions of the brain. But though mental processes as such cannot be rigidly localised the physiological machineries by which propositions can be expressed in spoken or written words and those which underlie their comprehension are localisable, though probably less sharply than less highly evolved functions. The rigid localisation which was for so long popular was based on the regular occurrence of specific disturbances in association with injuries of certain portions of the brain; that differently situated local lesions affect different elements of speech is incontestable, but, as Hughlings Jackson pointed out years ago, the localisation of a dis-order of speech does not justify the localisation of speech. The use of such terms as "centres," which implies sharply circumscribed structures, is inappropriate, but for clinical purposes the regions of the brain disease of which produces those disturbances of language that constitute the mani-festations of aphasia, may be referred to by the less definite term "area." These are restricted to the cerebral cortex and, in right-handed persons, lie in the left hemisphere of the brain. In about 50% of left handed persons speech is controlled by the right hemisphere. The concept of the strict lateralisation of all the functions involving the use of words may prove to be an over-simplification.

Around the auditory centre in the transverse gyri of the first temporal convolution there has developed a cortical mechanism, injury of which disturbs the comprehension of spoken speech and the recall of words (Fig. 38). When it is destroyed, the subject cannot understand spoken or

L

written language, or employ words with which to express his thoughts in either verbal utterance or writing. If the motor speech mechanism is not at the same time injured any attempt to speak results in mere jargon, or, if the disease is less severe, in the use of wrong or inappropriate words and in faulty grammatical construction. This is the *auditory speech area*. Its limits are indefinite, but it occupies a considerable portion of the middle and posterior parts of the first temporal gyrus. It is improbable that any subcortical masses of grey matter are concerned, but the normal activity of the auditory speech area naturally depends on its connections with other portions of the brain.

In the posterior part of the auditory speech area, extending as far occipitalwards as the angular gyrus, a portion of the cortex has evolved

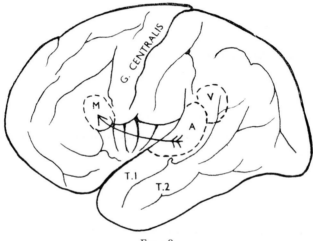

Fig. 38.

Diagram of the positions in the left hemisphere of the brain of the auditory *A.*, visual *V.*, and motor *M.*, speech areas. The arrow represents connections between the auditory and motor areas. The lips of the Sylvian fissure are separated to show the island of Reil.

functions to deal with visual speech symbols. This is the *visual speech area*. It is intimately connected with the visual areas of both occipital lobes. Theoretically injury of it results only in inability to read and write, but it is doubtful if such a pure visual aphasia ever occurs, the use and comprehension of articulate speech being almost invariably affected too, though in slighter degree.

Lesions of the left occipito-temporal lobe occasionally produce the condition known as *Pure Word Blindness*, the patient being unable to read written or printed words though he can converse naturally, understand spoken language and write correctly. This defect is not, however, part of an aphasia but the result of interruption of impulses of visual origin which have been differentiated and segregated in the occipital lobe on their way to more frontally placed association areas where they provide material for the elaboration of the visual elements of speech.

The motor speech area lies in Broca's convolution in the lower and posterior part of the left frontal lobe. This is not concerned in the innervation of the muscles of phonation and articulation, but in the elaboration of those movement patterns which underlie articulate speech. It is, in fact, a region in which representation of all movements of the larynx, tongue and lips, and of the thorax, which are employed in speech are combined into proper patterns. Certain subcortical structures, particularly part of the corpus striatum, are probably concerned in the rhythm and expression of voice.

Destruction of Broca's area results in speechlessness, but expletives and automatic expressions may at times be emitted. Since they do not as a rule represent propositions, they should not be regarded as elements of speech.

A special centre for writing has been postulated in the second left frontal convolution in front of the cortical representation of the movements of the hand and fingers, but there is no definite evidence of the existence of such a centre apart from that for acquired expert movements of the upper limb.

The separate portions of the cerebral cortex concerned in speech are intimately connected with one another and with other parts of the brain. Various diagrams have been constructed to represent these connections and the effects of interruption of them, and though such a materialistic attitude has been criticised there can be no doubt that as diagrams they are helpful in interpreting clinical symptoms. For instance, a lesion that severs the connections between the auditory speech area and Broca's gyrus, or isolates the latter, does not disturb seriously the comprehension of speech, but as word patterns which have been recalled in the temporal lobe cannot be transmitted to the motor speech area attempts to speak result in only unintelligible sounds, or in the utterance of disconnected or inappropriate words.

INVESTIGATION OF APHASIA

The complete investigation of any disturbance of speech is a long and time-consuming task, but the essential needs of clinical practice can usually be met by a short and concise examination. The more important facts that must be determined are:

1. Can the patient fully understand spoken language?
2. Can he use words?
3. Can he express his ideas accurately in words?
4. Can he read and understand what he reads?
5. Can he express himself in writing?

A fuller scheme of examination by which the nature and the degree of the defects can be more fully analysed is given below.

An examination must never be so prolonged that the patient tires, and aphasics tire rapidly under the strain of even short sittings; then responses to tests deteriorate and become unreliable and irregular. Short and repeated interviews are consequently advisable, particularly in complicated cases. Another reason is that speech, like other highly specialised but flexibly organised functions, is particularly labile and its efficiency is liable to vary under different conditions; even under the most favourable responses to tests are inconstant. A single examination may therefore fail to give a true picture of its state. Examination should also be conducted under as quiet and natural conditions as possible, with the patient free from distractions and anything that may divert his attention.

A simple record of a patient's responses to a series of tests will not alone give a complete account of his disability; this requires also a statement of the speed and readiness of response, and a classification of the mistakes that are made.

Fuller Examination.—Although the comprehension and formulation of word symbols is the basis of speech, it is for practical reasons advisable to determine first the power of utterance and enunciation of words, as, if expression by words is impossible, many of the following tests cannot be applied.

1. *Utterance of Words.*
   (1) Ability to utter simple words, less familiar words and words of several syllables. Extent of vocabulary.
   (2) Repetition of words spoken by the examiner.
   (3) The use of correct or incorrect words, or replacement by unintelligible sounds.
   (4) The omission or erroneous substitution of syllables.
   (5) Hesitations and inappropriate pauses in attempting to speak.
   (6) The rhythm and fluency of speech.

A patient who is apparently speechless may use words, as expletives and oaths, automatically, and may be able to sing the words of a song to its melody. The essential question is, if the words he can utter have a propositional value.

Tests.—The most satisfactory estimate of capacity can be obtained from spontaneous conversation if the patient is able to use words. Or he may be asked to describe how his illness commenced, his interests, his work or his mode of life.

If he cannot talk consecutively, he should be tested by replies to questions which he can understand, and by his power to repeat words and phrases.

2. *Comprehension of Articulate Speech.*—This is tested by noting the patient's response to spoken requests and commands. Tests should be arranged in order of increasing difficulty.

(1) He may first be asked to point to an object the name of which has been given to him.

(2) Questions and commands should first take the form of short sentences containing a single predicate, as "Close your eyes," "Place a hand on the top of your head," etc.

(3) They should then present a choice or selection, as "Place your left hand on the top of your head."

(4) Compound sentences may then be employed, as "Take that coin from the table and give it to me"; "Place one coin on the table, give me the second and keep the third in your hand."

(5) Finally, the response to complex sentences which contain in addition to the main clause two or more subordinate clauses, should be observed.

In cases of milder disorder of speech, failure of comprehension may be detected in ordinary conversation only, when the patient is not tuned up as he may be in formal tests.

3. *Recall and Formulation of Words.*—It should first be ascertained if the patient understands the nature and use of test objects which are employed in the examination to make sure that he does not suffer with an agnosia of objects as well as of words, and that his colour vision is intact.

(1) In the first place, he is asked to name familiar objects, as a knife, a key, a pencil, a coin, etc., and colours shown to him.

(2) His ability to recognise the significance of names may be tested by requesting him to point to or otherwise indicate objects the names of which are given to him.

(3) He may be asked to repeat the days of the week, the months of the year, the letters of the alphabet, or numbers in sequence.

(4) The ability to make use of other elements of speech can be ascertained by observing his replies to various questions in these and other tests, and in ordinary conversation.

4. *Expression of Thoughts and Ideas in Words.*—The next step should be to learn how far the patient can express his thoughts in speech. This can be best determined by noting attempts at ordinary conversation, if such attempts are possible.

(1) A request to describe what a picture or drawing represents is a useful test.

(2) If speech is more limited, examination may be restricted to replies to questions which require no more than simple affirmation or negation.

(3) Mistakes and defects may consist in the omission of necessary words, or the use of wrong or inappropriate words, in faulty grammatical structure of sentences, or merely in hesitations and pauses in conversation which is otherwise correct.

5. *Reading.*—Here, too, tests should be arranged in order of increasing difficulty, commencing with short words and simple phrases, and passing to longer and more complicated sentences.

(1) Cards on which names of familiar objects, or such commands as "Give me your hand," "Take this in your left hand," "Close your eyes and place your left forefinger on your nose," are inscribed in block letters or in easily legible script may be used.

(2) Later he may be tested by reading sentences of varying complexity, and explaining the meaning of what he has read.

(3) Reading aloud may reveal a defect in the translation of visual into auditory symbols which is not sufficient to disturb comprehension of whole sentences.

6. *Expression of Ideas in Writing.*

(1) The most useful measure of a patient's ability to express himself in writing is a letter he has written spontaneously, if one is available.

(2) Specific tests, as writing down the name of an object, or describing in writing a recent incident or a picture, may be employed.

(3) Writing to dictation reveals ability to translate auditory into visual symbols, but is applicable only when comprehension of speech is not seriously defective.

(4) Copying print into ordinary handwriting shows if the patient can substitute one form of visual symbols for another.

(5) The use of figures should also be investigated, as in addition and subtraction and in other arithmetic tests within the patient's educational level. Ability to calculate is often defective in aphasia, but may be lost apart from it.

If, owing to palsy of a hand, the patient is unable to use a pen or pencil, he may be asked to form words or short sentences by the proper arrangement of blocks or cards on which the individual letters are printed.

PHONATION AND ARTICULATION

The words of spoken language by which we express ourselves and communicate with others consist of large numbers of elementary sounds which are formed partly in the larynx, partly in the nasopharynx and mouth. In contrast to internal speech they are the product of purely mechanical processes dependent on the action of the musculature of the thorax, larynx, palate, tongue, lips and the lower jaw.

A current of air of sufficient force produced by expiration from the lungs is essential. Respiratory movements are automatic or reflex, but, though the same muscles are employed, those concerned in speech are voluntary and may be disordered though respiration is undisturbed. They determine the strength and are largely responsible for the rhythm of voice.

Phonation, or the production of vocal sounds, is a function of the larynx. The size and shape of the glottis and the tension and length of the vocal cords can be altered by action of the laryngeal muscles, and the rate and character of the vibrations transmitted to the column of air passing over them, and the sounds these aerial vibrations produce, can be by these means varied. These vocal sounds are, however, added to or modified as they pass through the nasopharynx and mouth, which act as resonating chambers, the form and size of which can be varied by movements of the soft palate, tongue, lips and lower jaw.

In other verbal sounds the larynx is not directly concerned; these are due to *articulation,* that is the production of vibrations in currents of air during their passage through the nasopharynx and mouth.

While vowels are mainly of laryngeal origin, consonants are formed chiefly by articulation. But this distinction is not absolute, for not only may vowels be modified in the supra-laryngeal air passages, but the proper enunciation of soft consonants as, B.W.T.V.Z., depends partly on phonation. Others, however, as P.T.K.S.F., are only articulated. The most useful classification of consonants for clinical purposes is into groups corresponding to the organs which are mainly concerned in their production, as labials, as P.B.M., linguals, as L.T., nasals, as M.N.NG.

Disturbance of Voice.—Paresis of respiratory movements sufficiently severe to affect voice seriously is rarely compatible with life, but when extensive it may enfeeble it, or disturb its regularity and rhythm. Stuttering, or a hesitancy or faltering in speech, often associated with involuntary repetition of letters, syllables or less differentiated sounds, is primarily due to spasms and inco-ordination of the respiratory muscles; it has generally a psychogenic basis.

Disturbances of phonation result from paresis of one or of both vocal cords; these can be observed directly by the laryngoscope. Total paralysis of both vocal cords causes complete aphonia, there is no voice and the patient can speak in whispers only. Voice is not lost when one vocal cord only is paralysed, as the healthy cord approximates to the middle line to narrow the glottis, but it becomes low pitched and hoarse. Abductor palsies cause little disturbance of the voice, but adductor paralysis, which is common in hysteria, produces aphonia.

The vocal cords play important parts in ordinary respiration too; they separate and widen the glottis during inspiration, but come nearer together in expiration. Inspiratory stridor often accompanies total bilateral abductor paralysis, and may occur in deep breathing when one cord only is affected.

Disturbances of articulation depend on whether all or some only of the movements concerned in it are disordered or lost. In ordinary bulbar palsy the lips, tongue and palate are usually affected together, but they may be involved separately. The vocal cords may be palsied too. Paralysis of the palate causes a nasal quality in the voice, as the posterior nares are not closed, and part of the vocal current consequently passes through the nose. Unilateral palsy of the tongue merely impairs the lingual consonants, but when bilateral the correct utterance of vibratives, as R., is impossible. When the lips are affected the labials, as P.B., are slurred or replaced by sounds resembling F. and V.

The disturbances of articulation which occur in bulbar palsy and result from lesions of bulbar motor nerves are associated with obvious paresis of the organs concerned and usually with wasting of their muscles. But disorders of phonation and articulation may be caused by supra-nuclear lesions which produce spastic paresis of the laryngeal and oral muscles. As the movements of the vocal cords, palate and tongue are habitually bilateral their muscles receive voluntary impulses from both sides of the brain, and their functions consequently suffer from bilateral cerebral lesions only. Then the vocal movements of the chest may be affected too, though ordinary respiration is unimpaired. As there is no wasting of the muscles of the tongue or lips, and as they may be employed in other movements, this has been termed *pseudobulbar palsy*. When severe it produces complete aphonia and anarthria, but if less severe speech may be merely characterised by slowness and hesitancy in the utterance of words, indistinctness or failure in the correct enunciation of certain sounds, and often by an explosive character—words uttered seem to be spat out.

Disorders of the extra-pyramidal system may also produce altera-tions of voice; it is often slow, feeble, low pitched and monotonous in Parkinson's disease, and tremulous, jerky or staccato in other affections. Inco-ordination of the vocal mechanisms, as occurs in cerebellar disease, tends to make utterance jerky and irregular in pitch and quality.

Examination.—Disorders of the apparatus of voice can be investigated directly. The movements of the vocal cords can be inspected by use of a laryngoscope, those of the palate, tongue and lips by direct observation.

Disturbances of phonation and articulation may occur separately or together. They are not easily distinguished by the inexperienced ear; a useful means of distinction is to ask the patient to whisper, which depends almost entirely on articulatory movements, and to hum with open mouth, which is practically pure phonation.

The special features of a dysarthria can be described in terms of the consonants which are not articulated correctly, as labial, lingual or nasal.

CHAPTER XVII

Agnosia and Apraxia

AGNOSIA

THE recognition of an object perceived by one of the senses is a complicated psychological process. It depends primarily on impulses transmitted from sense organs to receptive areas in the cerebral cortex where they excite a specific pattern, but it is also necessary that this sensory pattern should be combined or associated with the memory or mental images of the same or of a similar object which has been previously registered in the brain. It is not necessary that the mental image should correspond exactly with the perception of the new object, or contain representations of all its features; images stored in memory are particulate, that is, they consist of a number of parts each of which represents a feature of the object remembered. An unfamiliar breed of dog, for instance, is recognised as a dog as it presents to the senses certain characteristics which we associate with a dog. But recognition does not depend on synthesis of all the sense impressions derived from an object; the object is usually recognised as a whole, not as a sum of its parts. Even when homonymous hemianopia is present a familiar object is usually apprehended as a whole, though part of it lies within the blind portions of the fields of vision.

Failure to recognise an object may be due to insufficient or erroneous sense impressions; or it may be the result of loss of mental images, or engrams, of similar objects previously experienced; or of failure to link up the sense impressions it excites with these mental images owing to interruption of functional connections of different portions of the brain with one another.

When sense impressions are unimpaired and mental images are intact, inability to recognise objects perceived by one of the senses is known as *Agnosia*. It is due to failure to associate impressions immediately perceived with mental images based on earlier sensations derived from the same or from other sense organs.

Tactile Agnosia.—Inability to recognise familiar objects by touch or by handling, though they can be identified by vision and other senses, has been termed tactile agnosia, or more commonly astereognosis (p. 83). The term tactile agnosia is appropriate only when imperception is not due to defects in superficial or proprioceptive sensation, or to motor disabilities which prevent proper handling or exploration of the object.

Failure to recognise an object by touch and handling is, however, most commonly due to disturbances of sensation, owing to which the patient is not able to recognise accurately its physical properties, as its size, form, consistence and weight; in agnosia, on the other hand, these properties may be appreciated, but the object is not identified.

Visual Agnosia.—Owing to the highly organised state of visual perception and to the fact that it is by vision that objects are most commonly identified, visual agnosia is a more striking clinical condition. It consists in inability to recognise by sight objects and persons previously known, though there are no disturbances of visual acuity or changes in the fields of vision which can account for it. The patient sees the object and may be able to describe its features as perceived by vision, but he cannot identify it though familiar with it. When, however, the object is placed in his hand, or when he can explore it by touch, he recognises it at once. Similarly, the sight of a friend may give no clue to his identity, but he may be recognised at once by his voice when he speaks.

Occasionally there is an agnosia for certain objects only; pictures and drawings may have no significance, or there may be merely inability to recognise words, letters or other symbolic figures. The latter disturbance is closely related to aphasia, but in some cases it is not associated with other disorders of speech.

Visual agnosia is often combined with spatial disorientation (see p. 179) or spatial agnosia, or with defects of topographical memory or imagery, and sometimes with inability to describe familiar objects which are known chiefly by their visual features. Visual agnosia in any form is very rare and it is doubtful whether it ever occurs without accompanying gross loss of visual acuity, central or peripheral.

Corporeal Agnosia.—Agnosia may be limited to a patient's own body, and may take the form of failure to recognise the existence or identity of parts of it. For instance, he may be unable to recognise, name or indicate individual fingers on the affected hand, or to imitate with them movements displayed before him, though motion and sensation in them are intact.

More commonly corporeal agnosia takes the form of failure to recognise gross defects of function. It is, for instance, a common clinical experience that patients with complete homonymous hemianopia are unaware they are unable to see to one side until it is pointed out to them or they learn it by experience. A most striking example is the failure of a person blind as a result of bilateral cortical lesions to recognise his own blindness; he may insist he sees objects normally, and may even describe what he believes to be in front of him.

It frequently happens too that a patient with severe hemiplegia due to a cerebral lesion may not recognise that one side of his body is paralysed until it is demonstrated to him. This is more common when the left side is affected, probably as it may not be detected when accompanied by aphasia. If such a patient is asked to move one of his left limbs he may execute the movement by the corresponding right limb, apparently unaware of the error, and he may refer any sensory impression excited on the left side of the body to the corresponding point on the right side. The inability of many patients with recent partial hemiplegia to carry out by the affected limb movements which are actually possible till the limbs are brought within the range of vision or stimulated vigorously is often due to an agnosia or imperception of them; there is loss of memory of the existence of the affected side, it is forgotten or absent from consciousness. Even when the patient touches the paralysed arm or leg with his normal hand, he may not recognise it belongs to him, and may attempt to throw it aside as a foreign body. This condition may be associated with inability to distinguish the right and left sides of the body.

Unawareness of parts of the body, or of the existence of extensive disorders of function, may be accompanied by disturbances of sensation, but its occurrence without anæsthesia shows it cannot always be attributed to this. It must be regarded as a specific disorder due to interference with the body image. Each of us has a scheme or postural model of his body and of the spatial relations of its parts, that is, an image of the body as it exists, which is built up of past and present visual, tactile, postural and other sensory impressions. When a part of this scheme or image is injured the corresponding part of the body passes out of consciousness, the patient is no longer aware of it and does not recognise any disturbance within it: an agnosia exists.

Visual agnosia results from lesions in the posterior portion of the brain which interrupt connections between the visual centres and association areas; it occurs chiefly with disease of the left hemisphere of the brain, but in many cases wide-spread or even bilateral lesions are responsible for it. Corporeal agnosia is found with disease further forward in the parietal lobe, usually in its deeper portions, which interferes with the synthesis of cutaneous and proprioceptive impressions with other sensory data.

APRAXIA

Apraxia, which is a disorder of motor activities without paralysis or loss of movement, may be regarded as the motor counterpart of agnosia.

Many of our motor activities are innate or inherited, as those by which instinctive reactions are carried out; the patterns of these are inherent and fixed properties of the nervous system and some of them may be effected at subcortical levels. On the other hand, patterns of actions acquired during life, and particularly of those executed by means of tools and instruments, are developed gradually by learning; they are essentially cortical functions.

Between these two extremes are many activities, such as walking, that must be painfully acquired by the growing child but which are soon performed automatically, but none the less in response to volition.

A full understanding of the neural mechanisms underlying voluntary movement is not to be expected as the relationship between volition and neuronal physiology is necessarily obscure. In simple terms, however, the idea of the desired act or movement must be in some sense separate from the sensori-motor integration necessary for its completion. Failure to carry out such an act correctly may be due, at one end of the scale, to an intellectual defect which precludes formulation of the idea; to agnosia or inability to recognise the nature of the object to be used, or the method of its use; or to aphasia which prevents comprehension of an order to execute it; or, at the other end, to paralysis or ataxia of move-ment, or to loss of sensation of such severity that it interferes with the use of the limb. But even in the absence of intellectual disorders, of agnosia and of disturbances of motion and sensation, a person otherwise normal may be unable to carry out an act correctly though he recognises its nature and aim. This state, which is known as *Apraxia*, may be due to defect in the mental representation or conception of the act, to failure to evoke the necessary pattern or plan of movement, or to inability of the motor cortex to make use of the pattern of movement. As disturbances may occur in these different stages in the performance of a purposive act, apraxia may appear in various forms. It is essentially an inability to trans-late an aim or purpose into desired action.

In right-handed persons the physiological mechanisms which underlie the formulation of the idea of an act and the development of its pattern are focused in the lower and posterior part of the parietal lobe of the left hemisphere of the brain in the neighbourhood of the angular gyrus. There is no evidence of the existence of an eupraxic centre; the symptoms of apraxia, which occur with disease of this region, are due to interference with associational processes. The idea or conception of an act, which is a purely psychological function, can certainly not be restricted to any one circumscribed area of the cortex.

The nature and the distribution of manifestations of apraxia depend on the site of the lesion which determines them. Theoretically, when the left parietal lobe is injured apraxic symptoms appear on both sides of the body; when its connections with the left motor cortex are severed the right limbs only are involved; if its connections with the right hemisphere through the corpus callosum alone are interrupted, the symptoms are left sided.

But this simple scheme often fails to explain observations. Causal lesions are frequently multiple or diffuse, and division of the corpus callosum may not produce apraxia of the left limbs.

Ideational Apraxia is essentially a defect in the mental representation of the act, as a result of which the patient fails to evolve a proper plan of action. Simple and isolated movements may be unaffected, but more complicated actions with a definite end or purpose in view may be im-possible. In attempts to perform them spontaneously or to order the com-ponent movements are wrongly combined, some are omitted or replaced by unnecessary or incorrect movements, or an object, the nature of which is recognised by the patient, may be wrongly used. If given a toothbrush he may hold it correctly, and though he recognises its use he may brush his hair rather than his teeth with it.

The nature of the disturbance becomes more obvious in more complicated acts; when, for instance, the patient is asked to light a cigarette he may be unable to extract a match from the match-box, or, having succeeded in doing so, may attempt to strike it on the wrong side of the box, or he may insert the match instead of the cigarette in his lips, or after he has placed the cigarette there he may fail to light it. These errors in action are often prominent as the patient dresses; garments may be put on back to front, or trousers as a coat, and attempts to button them may fail.

Even simple acts, as protrusion of the tongue, may not be executed to command, though the patient may immediately afterwards lick his lips or bring out his tongue when asked to open his mouth. Imitation of simple movements is usually possible as the pattern is provided by vision, but it may fail in more complicated actions.

Ideational apraxia affects both sides of the body. It is generally the result of diffuse cerebral disease in which the posterior part of the left parietal lobe is particularly involved.

In *Ideomotor Apraxia* the idea or conception of the act is correctly formulated, but owing to interruption of association paths in the brain the pattern of the action fails to reach the motor centres. Consequently, though he knows how the act should be done the patient is unable to carry it out correctly; it seems as though he had forgotten how to do it.

The symptoms resemble those of ideational apraxia so closely that it is often difficult to distinguish them. It is chiefly in more purposive and complicated actions that the patient fails; his attempts to carry out a request are slow and confused, and perseveration, or senseless repetition of a movement recently performed when a new order is given, is common. These mistakes are more obvious in the execution of movements to order and in copying movements made in front of him than in his spontaneous activities. The response may be entirely wrong though the order is fully understood; he may, for instance, bring his finger to his nose when asked to touch his ear. Gestures to order, as beckoning, threatening, saluting, may be lost though used spontaneously. Simple instruments, as scissors or pen, cannot be employed accurately.

Ideomotor apraxia is usually distinguished from the ideational variety by its distribution. In right-handed persons only the right side of the body, and often only the arm, is affected when the lesion, which generally lies in the lower portion of the left parietal lobe, interrupts only connections to the left motor cortex. Theoretically a lesion in the anterior part of the corpus callosum, through which the pattern of action is transferred to the right hemisphere, should cause apraxia of the left limbs, and occasionally it does so, but it has been repeatedly found that its division has no such effect, or the left-sided apraxic disturbances are transient.

Constructional Apraxia.—This term has been applied to a condition in which there is no disturbance of ordinary movements, but the patient is unable to arrange objects or lines in a plan or pattern which is presented to him; he cannot copy drawings, arrange matches or build up a simple structure with a child's blocks. When he writes the words are incorrectly spaced and the directions of the lines are irregular. It is not in the use of objects that he fails, but in directing his movements according to a spatial plan furnished by vision or visual memories. Defects in the fields of vision, and visual disorientation and visual agnosia, must be excluded as possible factors.

Constructional apraxia is comparatively common and is seen in parietal lobe lesions, usually of the non-dominant hemisphere. Although appearing as a defect in performance it is clearly linked with failure of the normal perception of spatial relationships. In this respect it resembles apraxia for dressing and the two forms are often associated.

The curious neglect or denial of disability seen in parietal lobe lesions often declares itself in absurd excuses for inability to draw a simple figure.

Motor Apraxia or Innervation Apraxia.—It is doubtful if the condition which has been described under this name should be included in apraxia. The symptoms are always limited to one side of the body, usually to one hand. Large movements are awkward and inaccurate and finer movements, as writing, may be impossible. All types of movements are affected, even those which the patient is asked to copy. The essential feature is that the purpose or aim of any act that the patient attempts is always apparent, but its execution is defective. These disorders in motor performance have been attributed to inability of the motor cortex to make use of patterns of action owing to these failing to link up with kinæsthetic images derived from previous experiences, but frequently they can be equally well regarded as manifestations of inco-ordination of cortical motor activity, as a result of disorder of the sensory components which are essential to the planning and execution of purposive movement.

The symptoms of apraxia are frequently transient, and, as disturbances of other higher functions, they are often variable within short periods.

Examination of an Apraxic Patient

Disorders of motion, sensation and vision which may influence the responses to the tests should be carefully excluded, and if any disturbance of speech is present it should be ascertained if the patient can comprehend fully the task he is asked to do.

The limbs of each side of the body should be tested separately.

1. *Simple movements to order.*—Make a fist. Separate your fingers. Stamp your foot. Put out your tongue. Cough.

2. *Movements directed to parts of own body.*—Touch your nose. Place your hand on top of your head. Brush your hair with your hand. Place your right heel on your left knee.

3. *Symbolic acts.*—Beckon. Threaten. Throw a kiss. Salute.

4. *Purposive movements without objects.*—Show how you would knock on a door, ring a bell, use a key, turn the wheel of a barrel-organ.

5. *Purposive movements with objects.*—Brush your hair. Light a cigarette. Pour water into a glass and drink it. Tie a knot. Put on your coat.

6. *Imitation of movements performed before the patient.*

7. *Dressing.*—Put on a pair of gloves; a jacket presented with one sleeve inside out.

8. Draw a circle; put in the figures of a clock. Draw a house; a bicycle. Copy patterns in drawing or with matches or blocks.

Chapter XVIII

Neurology in Children

THE effects of disease on the developing nervous system and the causes of disease in the infant differ in many respects from those in the adult. Congenital malformations and cerebral damage in the perinatal period assume particular importance. Genetically determined disease, often involving recognised metabolic defects, are less common but emphasise the importance of an accurate family history. Infections may be both more insidious in their onset and more devastating in their effects. The difficulties of neurology in infants are undoubtedly due in part to relative neglect and ignorance of the functions and behaviour of the maturing brain.

Neurological investigation must be based on a knowledge of the expected normal. The new-born child moves its limbs spontaneously and expresses displeasure readily. The pupillary reactions to light and the corneal reflex are already present. The sucking reflex, a sign of grave disease in the adult, is of obvious biological value to the new-born. Below the age of three months other primitive reflexes are normally present. The grasp reflex is particularly strong in the few days after birth. Tonic neck reflexes may be obtained, the arm and sometimes the leg extending on the side to which the head is turned. In addition to these phenomena familiar from disease in the adult an important reflex is the rapid abduction of the arms in response to startle, either from noise or sudden change in posture.

Although there is some individual variation the absence of these reflexes below the age of three months or their persistence beyond this age is abnormal.

The plantar reflex does not assume its adult flexor form until the age of 2 years and is a valueless sign below that age. The tendon jerks do not differ significantly from those of the adult. Pædiatricians attach importance to the ease with which the knee jerk may be elicited by tapping the tibia rather than the patellar tendon as an indication of disease. This phenomenon is not, however, due to any enlarged reflexogenic zone but simply shows that only a minute stretch of the muscle is needed to elicit a phasic reflex. It is certainly a sign of hyperactive spinal reflex activity but its specificity cannot be compared to that of the Babinski reflex.

Signs of gross disease, paralysis, hypotonic or hypertonic limbs are easily recognisable, although their interpretation may prove difficult. Involuntary movements, apart from convulsions, are seldom seen in infancy and a condition that may later declare itself as athetosis presents simply as failure to use the affected limbs.

Apart from such obvious defects examination consists essentially of observing the rate of development of normal functions—the well known "milestones". A baby first smiles at about 6 weeks. At 4 weeks fixation of the eyes on a stationary object can be observed but a moving object is not followed until the age of three months. By this age some ability to support the head should be possible and at 24 weeks sitting with support. By 40 weeks the child should be able to sit unsupported and to stand holding on. Walking becomes possible at about 13 months and by this time the child should be able to express and understand a few words. A child of 2 should be running about actively, talking freely with a limited vocabulary, and should have control of the sphincters in the day time.

Visual acuity cannot be tested in the small infant beyond the ability to follow a moving object. Deafness is often overlooked and the child's failure to develop speech attributed to mental deficiency. Parents often insist that a child can hear when on examination no response can be detected to loud and meaningful noises.

The circumference of the head is a valuable clinical sign. Microcephaly is associated with many forms of mental deficiency. An abnormally large head, or even more significant, a rapidly increasing circumference, is an important indication of raised intracranial pressure. The normal range is:

Birth, 13 to $14\frac{1}{2}$ inches   12 months, 18 to 19 inches
3 months, 15 to $16\frac{1}{2}$ inches   18 months, $18\frac{1}{2}$ to $19\frac{1}{2}$ inches
6 months, $16\frac{1}{2}$ to $17\frac{1}{2}$ inches   24 months, 19 to 20 inches
9 months, $17\frac{1}{2}$ to $18\frac{1}{2}$ inches

The anterior fontanelle normally closes between the ages of 9 months and 2 years and the precise time of closure is not often important. It should be level with the cranial vault and is abnormal if it bulges or is sunken.

Beyond the age of 5 the symptoms of nervous disease rapidly approach those of the adult. Provided they are neither frightened or bored children of this age are easy to examine and, with a few notable exceptions, seldom attempt to mislead the examiner.

M

CHAPTER XIX

The Bladder and Rectum

*T*HE BLADDER.—The wall of the bladder contains unstriped muscle fibres arranged in various directions which together are known as the detrusor. Its contents are retained by tonic contraction of two sphincters at the proximal portion of the urethra. The internal sphincter, composed of unstriped muscle, is not essential in man: control of the bladder and of micturition remain possible after it has been damaged in the operation of prostatectomy. The external sphincter consists of striped muscle of the voluntary type.

The detrusor and the internal spincter are innervated by the pelvic splanchnic nerves, the external spincter by the pudendel nerves; both of these come from the second, third and fourth sacral segments of the cord.

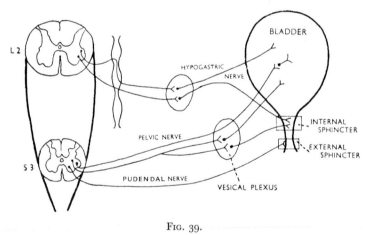

FIG. 39.
The nervous supply of the bladder and its sphincters.

The fibres of the pelvic nerves, which belong to the parasympathetic system, end in the vesical plexus and around ganglion cells in the wall of the bladder (Fig. 39). Short postganglionic units which take origin in these terminate in the muscular wall of the bladder and in its internal sphincter. Retention of urine owing to relaxation of the bladder and spasm of sphincter results from division of the pelvic nerves, but as the postganglionic units are capable of independent reflex activity retention may be later replaced by automatic evacuation.

Through the pudendal nerves, which belong to the somatic system, the external sphincter comes under voluntary control.

The bladder and its internal sphincter also receives sympathetic fibres from the upper lumbar segments of the cord through the hypogastric nerves and ganglia. These seem to be of little importance in man, as section of them may not disturb the storage or evacuation of urine. Afferent fibres enter the cord through both the pelvic and hypogastric nerves.

There is a reciprocal relation between the detrusor and the internal sphincter, as when contraction of the former reaches a certain intensity the latter relaxes and allows urine to escape into the urethra. Voluntary control is effected by tonic contraction of the external sphincter and by inhibition of the contractions of the wall of the bladder.

The tone of the detrusor keeps the bladder contracted down on its contents whether these are large or small in amount. But when intravesical pressure reaches a certain height, owing to accumulation of urine within the bladder, more or less rhythmic contractions of its walls develop. When these reach a certain intensity they lead to relaxation of the internal sphincter, escape of urine into the urethra and then, unless it can be successfully opposed by voluntary effort, to opening of the external sphincter and evacuation.

The amount of fluid the bladder can contain depends partly on the tone and reflex excitability of its muscle, partly on the rate at which it is introduced; larger quantities can be retained if introduced slowly, but when the intravesical pressure reaches about 50 cm. of water it causes discomfort, the rhythmic contractions become stronger and lead to relaxation of the sphincters.

Tension on its walls by fluid collecting within it is the physiological stimulus for contraction of the bladder. Its excitability may be increased by other agents, as exposure to cold, certain sounds, and emotional and psychological factors. A sudden increase of intra-abdominal pressure, as that produced by coughing and straining, may also augment intravesical pressure and cause vigorous contraction of the detrusor.

On the other hand, frequent or prolonged distension owing to obstruction in the urethra, or loss of tone in its walls as occurs in tabes dorsalis, reduces the reflex excitability of the detrusor and allow excessive amounts of urine to collect within the bladder.

The most serious disturbances of vesical function are those that result from acute injuries of the spinal cord and of the cauda equina. The immediate effects are almost identical whether the sacral segments or their roots are involved, or the lesion lies higher in the cord. The detrusor becomes at once toneless and fails to respond by contraction when stretched by accumulating urine, and as the internal sphincter remains contracted *retention* results. The bladder then behaves like a semi-elastic bag; when it cannot be further distended intravesical pressure may force the sphincters and *dribbling incontinence* occurs. As the external sphincter is also paralysed and toneless voluntary control is also lost.

If fluid is introduced gradually into such a bladder the intravesical pressure rises slowly, and when it has attained a certain level remains unchanged if no more fluid is introduced. In the normal bladder, on the other hand, the rise of pressure is more rapid, but it falls quickly if the amount of fluid remains unaltered, since by virtue of the tone of its muscular walls it adapts itself quickly to the bulk of its contents (Fig. 40).

It is in this stage that the danger of infection of the paralysed bladder is greatest. The tonelessness of its walls and the absence of spontaneous contractions permits infected material to collect in pockets and dependent parts from which it cannot easily be removed, more particularly as it is never fully evacuated either by dribbling incontinence or by irrigation. Penetration of infection into its walls excites inflammatory reactions which

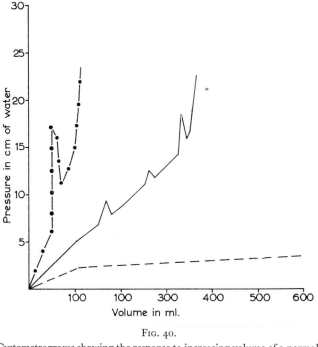

FIG. 40.

Cystometrograms showing the response to increasing volume of a normal bladder (————), an atonic bladder (– – –) and a hyperexcitable bladder (– · – · –).

impede recovery of tone, and as secondary fibrosis is liable to occur if it is neglected the bladder may become permanently contracted.

If, however, the bladder escapes serious infection signs of recovery appear as shock passes off. The detrusor regains tone, as is shown by increasing resistance to distension and by a greater capacity to adapt itself to the bulk of its contents; it is no longer a passive reservoir. Later, rhythmic contractions similar to those which occur in the normal state appear, and when they reach a certain intensity the internal sphincter relaxes and permits escape of urine. This *reflex or automatic micturition* is usually independent of extrinsic stimuli, but may be excited by anything which increases intravesical tension, as straining, pressure on the abdomen, or spasm of the abdominal walls.

A bladder may develop reflex automatism even when its connections with the central nervous system are interrupted, as by destruction of the cauda equina or of its spinal centres in the sacral segments. This depends on the independent activity of the vesical plexus and of the post-ganglionic autonomic cells and fibres in its walls. It is not, however, under voluntary control, its capacity is less than normal, and as a rule it does not empty itself fully.

Though in the early stages there is no essential difference between palsy of the bladder due to destruction of the sacral segments or of the cauda equina and that which results from higher spinal lesions, in the latter case recovery of automatic evacuation is more rapid and its response to distension is brisker. On the other hand, when the sacral segments are destroyed the external sphincter may remain toneless and dribbling incontinence is more likely to be the final result. When sensory impulses from its walls are not interrupted in the hypogastric nerves or in the spinal cord, the discomfort due to over-filling of the bladder induces voluntary efforts to empty it by contraction of the abdominal and relaxation of the perineal muscles.

Voluntary control of bladder function appears to depend on the integrity of the cortex of the orbital surface of the frontal lobes and of fibres in close anatomical relationship to the spinothalamic tracts in the spinal cord. Retention of urine may occur in the stage of shock in acute hemiplegia but does not persist. Incontinence is common in diffuse cerebral disease with dementia and also in more localised disease of the frontal lobes. This often consists more of socially undesirable but voluntary emptying of the bladder rather than loss of sphincter control.

In slowly progressive or partial lesions of the spinal cord, not causing shock, the usual sequence is difficulty and delay in starting micturition which may lead to retention, and later incontinence of the dribbling type from the over-filled bladder, or the development of reflex micturition.

When, however, the reflex excitability of the bladder is high, as it may be when there is a spastic paresis of the lower limbs, *urgency* or *precipitancy of micturition* is a common sympton; the contractions of its walls become so vigorous they cannot be resisted by the external sphincter and urine escapes suddenly, usually in large amounts.

THE RECTUM

The smooth muscles of the walls of the rectum are innervated by sympathetic fibres which pass through the upper lumbar roots and the hypogastric nerves, and by parasympathetic fibres from the third and fourth sacral segments which reach it through the pelvic nerves. The internal sphincter, which consists of unstriated muscle, has a similar nervous supply, but the external sphincter, which is composed of striated muscle, is innervated by the pudendal nerve which takes origin in the lower sacral segments. Afferent impulses enter the cord through the pelvic and pudendal nerves.

As in the bladder, a reciprocal relation exists between the rectum and its sphincters; when the rectum contracts the sphincters tend to relax. The adequate stimulus for defæcation is stretching of the walls of the rectum by fæcal matter collecting within it; when this reaches a certain degree rhythmic contractions develop and the internal sphincter relaxes, but the external sphincter, which is under voluntary control, may for a time prevent the escape of fæces. The parasympathetic system plays a more important part in defæcation than the sympathetic; the latter probably only tends to inhibit movements of the bowel in order to permit accumulation of its contents. In man section of the hypogastric nerves has little effect, and even when the parasympathetic system is injured by disease of the sacral segments of the cord, of the cauda equina or of the pelvic nerves, automatic defæcation is possible through the agency of a peripheral plexus. As impulses to the external sphincter by way of the pudendal nerves are usually interrupted at the same time, voluntary control is no longer possible. Defæcation is also aided by contraction of the perineal muscles, especially of the levator ani.

Acute lesions of the spinal cord involving either the sacral segments or higher levels depress the tone and the rhythmic contractions of the rectum. As the sphincters are for a time toneless too, fæcal incontinence may occur owing to passive flow of fæces along the bowel, especially after administration of a purgative, but if the fæces are solid there is usually obstinate constipation. When a finger is inserted into the anus its sphincters are found to be lax, and though they may contract momentarily owing to local stimulation, they rapidly dilate again. The *anal reflex*, which consists of a tonic contraction of the sphincter on stroking or pricking the skin in the region of the anus, cannot be obtained.

In diseases of longer standing the rectum and its sphincters regain tone and some reflex activity: this is apparently due to a peripheral nervous plexus. When the lesion lies above the sacral centres some degree of reflex recovery is more likely than when these are injured. Owing to sluggish reaction of the bowel and tonic contraction of the sphincters constipation is more common than incontinence, but precipitant evacuation may occur, especially when the fæces are fluid or when the bowels are stimulated by a purgative, or as a result of a sudden increase of intra-abdominal pressure, as that produced by straining or coughing.

SEXUAL FUNCTION

Impotence and failure of ejaculation are inevitable if the pelvic para-sympathetic nerves, the sacral roots or the sacral segments of the spinal cord are destroyed. Impotence is also common in chronic or progressive spinal cord disease but even when there has been complete cord transection reflex erection of the penis may occur.

In the absence of other definite symptoms or signs of organic disease impotence is almost certainly psychogenic.

CHAPTER XX

The Autonomic System

INNERVATION of visceral organs and glands, which is among the chief functions of the autonomic system, scarcely concerns the neurologist directly, but other functions, particularly control of the peripheral blood vessels, sweating and pilomotor reactions, may be affected by disease of both its central and peripheral nervous portions and the disorders which result may be valuable symptoms in neurological diagnosis. Disturbances in the innervation of certain plain muscles, particularly of those supplied by the cranial and sacral autonomic systems, also come into the domain of the neurologist.

The peripheral autonomic system is distinguished from the somatic peripheral nervous system by the fact that all its fibres which leave the central nervous system end in peripheral ganglia, and relays of fibres from these connect them with their peripheral organs: no autonomic fibre from the brain-stem or cord reaches a peripheral organ directly.

The two divisions of the autonomic system are distinguished by their anatomical relations and by their reactions to chemical substances.

Sympathetic fibres take origin in the lateral columns of the grey matter of the spinal cord between the first thoracic and second lumber segments, pass out in the ventral roots as fine medullated fibres, known as white rami, and end in lateral or more peripherally placed ganglia. In the lower portion of the system there is one sympathetic ganglion to each spinal root, but the upper three ganglia are fused into the stellate ganglion. All these are connected by the sympathetic chain which consists of white rami that run up and down between ganglia before they reach those in which they end. The cervical segments do not give origin to sympathetic elements, but fibres from the upper thoracic segments run upwards in the cervical sympathetic trunk to the inferior and superior cervical ganglia, fibres from which innervate blood vessels, sweat and other glands, and plain muscles of the orbit and of the hair follicles of the head, face, upper limbs and the upper part of the thorax.

The fibres which arise in the central nervous system are known as preganglionic. Post-ganglionic fibres, which take origin from the cells of the sympathetic ganglia, join somatic nerves and blood vessels, and through them are distributed to their peripheral destinations.

The pre-ganglionic fibres of each ventral root may reach several ganglia above or below the level of their exit. Post-ganglionic fibres have a more restricted distribution.

The *parasympathetic* system is related to the brain-stem and the sacral segments of the cord. Its pre-ganglionic fibres enter the third, seventh,

168

ninth and tenth cranial nerves, and the pelvic nerves by way of the second and third sacral roots. All these fibres end by synapses around ganglion cells in the vicinity of the organs to which they carry impulses; the post-ganglionic fibres are consequently short and often form plexuses at or near their terminations. The parasympathetic supply of the un-striated muscles of the ciliary body and of the iris, and the sacral inner-vation of the bladder and rectum, are described in the chapters in which the physiology and pathology of these organs are dealt with.

The chemical transmitter in all autonomic ganglia is acetylcholine. Post-ganglionic parasympathetic fibres also secrete acetylcholine at their

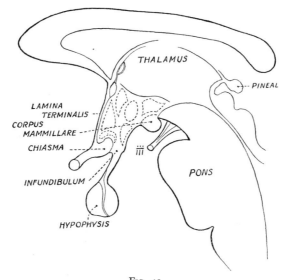

FIG. 41.

Diagram of the hypothalamus and of some of its intrinsic nuclei (after Le Gros Clark).

termination. Most sympathetic post-ganglionic fibres liberate nor-adrenaline but those to sweat glands are said to be cholinergic. It has recently become clear that the response to autonomic innervation depends not only on the nature of the chemical transmitter but also on the type of receptor in the effector organ.

A common sensory mechanism serves both the somatic and autonomic systems. Afferent fibres which convey visceral sensation and subserve autonomic reflexes run centralwards through splanchnic and other auto-nomic nerves, those from the skin and subcutaneous structures in somatic nerves and along the coats of blood vessels. They eventually reach a spinal or corresponding cranial ganglion where their cells of origin are situated. Proximal branches of these cells carry impulses through the dorsal roots to the central nervous system.

The hypothalamus, the grey matter lining the ventral portion of the wall of the third ventricle, extends from the lamina terminalis to the anterior end of the mid-brain (Fig. 41). Its total weight is about 4 g. and yet it controls an astonishing variety of vital functions concerned with adjustment to changes in external environment or in the milieu interieur. The numerous hormones of the anterior lobe of the pituitary are each controlled by a specific liberating hormone secreted in the hypothalamus and passing down the pituitary stalk.

The extremely complex mechanisms involved in maintaining a constant body temperature range from involuntary and unconscious vasomotor changes, sweating and shivering, to man's conscious adaptation of his external environment. All appear to depend on a small group of neurons in the hypothalamus sensitive to changes in temperature and linked with the efferent flow to the autonomic centres in the brain-stem.

Appetite and all that it implies in the control of metabolism is similarly dependent on neurons sensitive to changes in blood glucose. The reabsorption of water from the renal tubule is controlled by the anti-diuretic hormone of the posterior lobe of the pituitary gland, also under hypothalamic control.

The clinical study of hypothalamic disorders is hampered by the minute quantities of neuro-hormones involved and the inaccessability of the organ. Only gross disturbances can occasionally be recognised, of which the commonest is diabetes insipidus resulting from destructive lesions of the posterior pituitary or its hypothalamic connections. Failure to secrete the anti-diuretic hormone causes severe polyuria and thirst. Obesity, disorders of sexual development and of the natural sleep rhythm may occasionally be attributed to hypothalamic lesions.

The hypothalamus, in addition to its controlling humoral mechanisms, is also to some extent influenced by the cerebral cortex, particularly that of the orbital surface of the frontal lobes from which fibres also probably reach lower autonomic centres directly.

Regulation of the temperature of the body by alterations in the flow of blood through the smaller vessels and by exciting or arresting sweating, is the chief function of the sympathetic fibres distributed to the skin. Stimulation of a ventral root which contains sympathetic fibres causes vaso-constriction and sweating on the corresponding dermatome, but section of a single root may produce no symptoms as there is an extensive overlap from adjacent roots. Owing to their more restricted distribution, division of post-ganglionic fibres in a peripheral nerve leads to dilatation of blood vessels and abolishes sweating in its cutaneous area.

Stimulation of sympathetic fibres also excites by contraction of the erectores pilorum erection of hairs and prominence of hair follicles, and increases the supply of sebum which keeps the skin greasy and soft, for when the muscles of the hair follicles contract they compress the sebaceous glands and extrude their secretion. Section of post-ganglionic fibres consequently leads to dryness of the skin and absence of pilomotor reactions.

The local response to change in temperature is unaffected by loss of the afferent nerve supply as the receptor organs are not those locally in the limbs but are in the hypothalamus and respond to a change in temperature in the blood.

Mechanical stimuli also influence the flow of blood through cutaneous vessels. This depends on an axon reflex in which the impulse does not reach the central nervous system but both the afferent and efferent limbs of the reflex arc are formed by branches of a single axon.

Local symptoms of autonomic dysfunction due to lesions of the spinal cord or peripheral nervous system are seldom obtrusive. Interruption of post-ganglionic vaso-motor and sudo-motor fibres causes initial flushing of the distal segments of the limb and sweating is absent. The denervated end-organs soon become hypersensitive to circulating adrenaline and the hand is then paradoxically cold and pale. There will naturally be no response to thermal stimulation of other parts of the body as the response through the hypothalamus cannot act if the efferent nerve supply is lost.

The effect of pre-ganglionic lesions is similar but less pronounced owing to their wide distribution and extensive overlapping. The hyper-sensitivity of the denervated end organs may be delayed and less severe.

The axon reflex responsible for the spreading flare around minor skin trauma is abolished in skin anæsthetic because of a lesion of a peripheral nerve, but is retained if the injury is in the dorsal root. This is sometimes of value in distinguishing traumatic lesions of the brachial plexus from avulsion of the cervical roots.

After transection of the spinal cord the temperature of the skin below the corresponding level is no longer adjusted by alterations in the flow of blood through its vessels in response to heat or cold. In man also an acute transverse lesion of the cord is followed by diminution of the temperature of the skin of the paralysed parts when they are exposed, but at first it may be warmer owing to depression by shock of the vaso-constrictors. A zone of hyperæmia is occasionally visible at the level corresponding to the lesion. When thoracic segments are injured the temperature of the lower limbs fails to respond to immersion of an arm in warm or cold water, but warming or cooling a leg excites the character-istic reaction above the level of the lesion as it is determined by the temperature of the blood acting on higher centres, not on afferent im-pulses. The vessels of the paralysed limbs respond normally to local thermal and mechanical stimuli.

Slowly progressive spinal disease produces less disturbance as the sympathetic system can to some extent adjust itself to gradually changing conditions. Extensive damage of the lateral column of grey matter of the cord, as may occur in syringomyelia and poliomyelitis, causes symptoms similar to those which result from division of pre-ganglionic fibres.

The most striking and extensive disturbances of the vaso-motor system are seen after acute destruction of the first and second thoracic segments; the skin of the whole body becomes cold and blue, the rectal temperature may fall to 80° F., the pulse rate and respiratory movements are abnormally slow, the secretion of urine is diminished and metabolism reduced to a very low level.

In hemiplegia the state of the cutaneous vessels, and consequently the temperature of the skin on the paralysed side, varies: the limbs are sometimes warmer, sometimes colder than the normal, but the vaso-motor responses remain undisturbed. The more usual coldness of the limbs is due mainly to inactivity or disuse.

Many of the phenomena which have been termed "trophic," or attributed to affection of special systems of fibres or to vaso-motor disturbances, are a result of disuse rather than of nervous lesions. When a limb is immobilised by splinting, by palsy, or by a painful state, the blood flow through it decreases, and as a result the skin atrophies, loses its normal wrinkles and elasticity, is usually colder than normal, becomes more vulnerable and heals more slowly. Subcutaneous tissues and even bone may atrophy too. As the vessels become more permeable œdema results, and the limb may be cyanotic owing to loss of the pumping action of the muscles. These changes are due to diminished and reduced metabolism in the tissues, not to disturbances in the autonomic system; the blood vessels respond to local stimuli and to variations in the temperature of other parts.

Sweating also depends on the integrity of post-ganglionic fibres; these are however, cholinergic, though they accompany the ordinary sympathetic outflow from the spinal cord and run with sensory peripheral nerves. It is closely related to, though not dependent on, vaso-motor activity: the main function of both is the regulation of temperature.

Sweating may be induced by external heat, or by the administration of hot drinks, or by drugs as aspirin. Pilocarpine acts directly on the glands and may cause sweating after degeneration of all their nervous connections. A rise of temperature causes sweating mainly on the trunk, head and neck, while exertion and emotion excites it first on the palms and soles.

Degeneration of post-ganglionic fibres abolishes sweating in the area of their distribution, and the skin becomes dry and often scaly. It is more obvious when general perspiration is induced, and can be made visible by dusting with a powder which adheres to the sweating areas, or with a mixture of starch and iodine which becomes blue where moistened by sweat.

Division of pre-ganglionic fibres also reduces secretion of sweat, but it is usually obvious only when fibres issuing out of several ventral roots are divided, as where they are collected together in the cervical sympathetic chain, or when a lateral horn of grey matter is extensively damaged.

After a sudden transverse lesion of the cord those parts below its level are usually at first dry, but later the skin may become moist, and profuse sweating can often be induced by local stimuli, particularly by those which excite flexor spasms, as stroking a sole, pinching a leg, passing a catheter, or by heat. Sweating is less affected by slowly progressive lesions, but if the observer draws his fingers upwards along the trunk, the softer and moister impression received from the skin above the level of the disease can often be recognised. This is often a useful sign in the localisation of spinal disease.

Pronounced disturbances of sweat secretion may result from lesions of the lateral part of the medulla and pons, where there is probably a relay station in the path from the hypothalamus. The face and neck of the same side and the opposite half of the body remain dry when sweating is provoked by heat or exercise, but can be excited by local stimuli as the peripheral nervous supply of the sweat glands remains intact.

Occasionally a local outbreak of sweat is caused by stimuli that do not ordinarily evoke it. It occurs most commonly on some part of the face or neck, and is generally most pronounced during mastication. It may be a congenital abnormality; when acquired it is probably due to sympathetic fibres which had been divided by operation on the neck or by disease developing abnormal connections during regeneration.

The Pilomotor System.—Pilomotor reactions can be elicited by local stimuli, as a tap, which act directly on the muscles of the hair follicles, or reflexly by moving contacts, tickling, a prick or pinch, a cold object or a Faradic current. The erection of hairs and the appearance of cutis anserina are at first seen only at and immediately around the spot that is stimulated, but they spread slowly and often widely; the application of a cold object to the skin may cause an extensive, even a general reaction. These reactions are restricted to the side which is stimulated, but are not easily elicited in certain regions, as the face, head and hands. A pilomotor response on the same side of the trunk and on the limbs can often be obtained by pinching a trapezial fold, but it is a capricious reaction and may not appear in many parts.

Local reactions are abolished by injuries of peripheral nerves which contain post-ganglionic fibres, but pre-ganglionic lesions have little influence on them. The latter abolish more widespread reactions, as those due to cooling another part of the body and to emotional stimuli.

The pilomotor reflex is generally lost for a time below the level of an acute spinal lesion, but usually it reappears, and may be exaggerated when the paralysed limbs become spastic. In spastic hemiplegia the reaction is often excessive on the paralysed side.

Both goose skin and sweating are often excessive in tender and painful areas, provided the post-ganglionic fibres to the area are not injured.

CHAPTER XXI

Mental State

ALTHOUGH a complete assessment of the mental state of his patient, such as is required by a psychiatrist, is not usually necessary for the neurologist, it is important he recognises its main traits and the nature of any deviations from the normal it may present. For, in the first place, the reliability of the history of his illness, the importance of which has already been emphasised, depends largely on the patient's memory, on his attitude towards it, and on his power and facility in expressing his ideas. In the second place, mental symptoms often result from organic disease of the brain, and neurological disturbances may occur in, or develop during the course of, a disorder that is primarily psychological. As all mental processes depend on the activity of the brain, which may be, in Shakespeare's word, regarded as "the forge and working-house of thought," a divorce of neurology and psychiatry is theoretically artificial and inadvisable, though frequently made in practice.

Speculation on the anatomical substrate of the mind has engaged the attention of philosophers but a mastery of their arguments is not required for the practice of clinical neurology. It may be assumed for practical purposes that both cortical and subcortical structures are involved in mental processes. Consciousness, at least, may depend on an effect of the reticular formation in the brain-stem in "alerting" the entire cerebral cortex. Such a hypothesis is compatible with the profound mental effects sometimes observed in lesions confined to the mid-brain and also with the obvious importance of the cerebral cortex as a whole in the processes of thought.

No attempt will be made here to discuss the nature of mental processes and their abnormalities; the intention of this chapter is to deal only with those modifications and disorders of mind that may be associated with disease of the brain, or with other conditions which present neurological symptoms. The more important of these are impairment of consciousness, alterations in mood and temperament, disturbances of memory and of attention, disorientation in time and space and abnormal suggestibility.

State of Consciousness.—The degree of awareness of surroundings and the responsiveness to external stimuli varies even in normal health. In deep *coma* the patient cannot be roused, the corneal and pupillary reflexes may be absent, muscle tone and the stretch reflexes are frequently abolished, and few responses can be obtained by stimulation. In milder degrees reflex activities, including those of the pupil, swallowing and the corneal reflexes, may be present, and the patient may react to painful stimuli, but no sign of consciousness can be elicited. The term *stupor* is applied to states of partial loss of consciousness from which the patient can be wakened, but into which he tends to relapse. In it movements of the voluntary type are absent or rare, but there is often a tendency to resist interference and to catalepsy, that is, to keep portions of the body, and particularly the limbs, in attitudes in which they are placed passively. *Confusion* is a milder degree of defect of consciousness; it is generally accompanied by disorientation in time and place.

Intelligence.—The neurologist rarely requires an actual measurement of intelligence, as determination of an intellectual quotient, but an estimate of his patient's intellectual level, and of general or specific defects in it, is often important in the investigation of organic disease of the brain. Such an estimate must naturally take into account the subject's education and professional level, his experiences and his opportunities for intellectual and social development.

Deterioration of intellectual capacity, which often results from injury or disease of the brain, may assume different forms, but the most essential are those which lead to changes in conduct or behaviour, and in the capacity to carry on social relations and business affairs to which the patient has been previously accustomed. As observation and questioning of the patient and his companions usually give sufficient information, special tests are rarely necessary.

In progressive failure or dissolution of mind all intellectual activities generally suffer, but the more complex, the more abstract and the least firmly organised deteriorate earlier and more severely than the simple, the more automatic and the most organised. The more complex and comprehensive a task or problem, the less is the chance of its correct performance or solution. While familiar acts which had become more or less automatic may be possible, the patient may be incapable of dealing with new problems, though they are within the scope of persons of his age and education. This is especially so when they require reasoning, planning or working from past experiences. It is, however, particularly in dealing with abstract subjects, as calculating, grasping the significance of stories or of conversation, and of solving problems that failure is most likely. Judgment is often defective, and initiative and decision lacking. The mode of response may be as significant as failure in performance; the time and rate of reaction are lengthened, and tasks are attempted or solved in a round-about manner.

In more severe degrees of intellectual impairment the patient tires quickly in mental tasks, and then performance deteriorates rapidly. Even comprehension of ordinary conversation is retarded, and failure to link up immediate impressions with past experiences results in inability to seize meanings. There may consequently be a certain amount of confusion and disorientation in time and space. This condition is frequently met in mild degrees of dementia associated with organic disease of the brain, as in general paralysis, arterio-sclerotic degeneration and intracranial tumours. It occurs also in certain poisonings and in post-epileptic states.

Mood.—Marked changes in mood are less prominent in organic cerebral disease, but when present they may throw light on symptoms of which a patient complains, and must be taken into account in the evaluation of his disabilities. An elated or euphoric person may minimise or neglect his symptoms; a depressed or anxious patient tends to exaggerate them. From the dull and apathetic patient little information can be obtained without prolonged questioning; the excitable or self-absorbed person describes every symptom at length, and recurs repeatedly to them after the subject has been changed. The behaviour of the neurasthenic who brings long lists and descriptions of his complaints and discusses them in wearisome detail is the antithesis of that of the patient suffering with organic disease who usually states his symptoms in a few words, and often seems more concerned with their cause than with his disabilities. In the hysterical patient too there is as a rule an apparent, and probably real, unconcern over his symptoms.

Endogenous depression, although almost certainly the result of a biochemical disorder of the brain, is still regarded as the province of the psychiatrist. As it can be cured it is extremely important to recognise that most such patients present with symptoms that could equally be due to accepted forms of organic disease, such as early morning headache. Few complain spontaneously of depression but, if directly questioned, nearly all will admit at once that they are deeply depressed. The classical insomnia, anorexia and torpor are inconstant symptoms and the diagnosis must often be made in their absence.

Unnatural anxiety is a more common feature of the psychoneuroses than of organic disease. The patient is obsessed by fears and doubts that are usually vague and apparently causeless, but anxiety may accompany any serious illness of the nature of which the patient is aware, and, if of a nervous temperament, even insignificant symptoms may excite undue apprehension. The reaction to emotional or affective stimuli, particularly to those related to his state, is generally exaggerated. Anxiety is usually combined with some degree of depression.

A patient with organic cerebral disease not uncommonly lacks insight into his condition, though its seriousness is obvious to others. Sometimes his attitude is one of indifference or of unwarranted cheerfulness, even though he suffers severely.

Lack of inhibition and too free association of ideas may result in inappropriate facetiousness and irrelevant witticisms, often of a coarse nature, and may be accompanied by unrestrained or childish behaviour, as micturition in public or sexual improprieties. This state may alternate with periods of dullness, apathy and lack of spontaneity, or with phases of excitement.

Emotional instability, or alteration in temperament and character, may also result from structural damage of the brain. Pathological emotional display, as apparently causeless outbursts of laughter or tears, which is a common symptom in pseudobulbar and bilateral spastic palsies, may or may not be accompanied by corresponding emotion.

Memory.—Memory depends on a series of physiological and psychological processes which extend between perception of a stimulus and its recall or reproduction in mind.

In the first place, it is necessary that the impression should be perceived, though it is not essential that its nature or all its details should be apprehended, and that it should then be combined or linked with mental relics of past experience which endow it with meaning or significance. Most of the impressions we receive are fleeting, and soon pass beyond recall; to serve for memory it is necessary that they are fixed and retained in some form. This depends on several factors: their emotional content and interest are particularly important; the more vivid the emotional reaction it excites the more likely is the impression to serve as stuff for memory, though unpleasant experiences may be suppressed or at least kept below the level of consciousness. Attention is even more important; only that small proportion of the innumerable and multifarious stimuli we encounter in daily life which attracts attention is perceived in such a form that it can be stored up for recall. If at the time of their occurrence they fail to excite attention because it is lacking or otherwise occupied, they do not readily become subjects for memory. Retention depends on other factors too; repeated recall of an impression or idea, or its close association with circumstances which frequently come into consciousness, makes retention firmer and more permanent. This explains the greater liability of memory of recent happenings to fail in many pathological conditions than of those of the more distant past, which have become more firmly fixed by repeated recall.

The recall and reproduction in mind of impressions previously experienced is a psychological process the nature of which, as of many other psychological activities, is not fully understood. Many memories seem to recur automatically; for no apparent reason a vision or memory of the past may suddenly appear more or less vividly in mind, or we may recall an event of the past by voluntary effort. In most circumstances, however, we remember by association; an immediate happening wakes a chain of associations with one of which the event was originally linked up, and it is then reproduced in consciousness. Sometimes this association is direct; we may fail to recall the features of a face or a picture, but remember it accurately when we see it again, and a sentence from a paragraph or a line of a poem eludes us till we hear or recall the initial words. At other times it is less direct or obscure.

Loss of memory of events actually perceived may therefore be due to failure of fixation, of retention or of recall. Fixation may fail owing to lack of interest or attention to it at the time of its happening; it may not

N

then appear to concern us, or our attention may be occupied by other events. When absorbed by work or interests, we may fail to remember where we have placed an object. This is a more or less normal happening, especially in advanced years and when we are tired, and it occurs in many psychological and pathological states. Failure to retain memory pictures may also be due to isolation of the event or idea so that it does not fit into a series or frame, or to the absence of its recall over long periods of time.

Recall is disturbed by disorders of the psychological processes by which it is normally evoked, or of physiological processes which are the basis of the operations of these faculties of mind.

There may be failure of memory for either the whole or part of the past; or the loss may be of either recent or more remote events. In Korsakoff's syndrome, for example, what happened in the distant past may be accurately recalled, though there is no memory of recent happenings. Islands of memory may, however, persist within a period of amnesia. The amnesic patient is frequently not aware of his loss of memory, and may attempt to fill up the blanks by phantasies or imaginary happenings which are often described with remarkable conviction.

Injuries of the head and acute cerebral lesions, especially such as cause loss of consciousness, usually produce loss of memory for a period more prolonged than that of unconsciousness. Patients who have had cerebral concussion often say they were unconscious during hours or days when, according to independent evidence, they were more or less fully aware of their surroundings. The length of amnesia may be employed as an indication, though not an accurate measure, of the severity of an injury when the duration of unconsciousness is not definitely known.

Frequently a patient is unable to recall how an accident happened, or the events which led up to it. This retrograde amnesia may extend for days and even weeks prior to the accident. As recovery advances memory returns gradually, first for more distant, later for events immediately before the accident; but frequently recovery is patchy, that of certain incidents or periods reappearing within a period of complete amnesia. Sometimes after recovery blanks or lacunæ persist permanently.

The state of memory can be estimated by questioning and by observation during examination. The capacity for fixing and retaining impressions, which is often affected by physical disease that may not influence memory of the past, can be tested by asking the patient to repeat a series of words or numbers either spoken or written, to repeat a short statement or story, or to describe a picture or drawing shown him a few minutes earlier.

Attention.—The importance of attention in investigations in which the co-operation of the patient is necessary has been emphasised, and the part it plays in supplying material for memory of the past and comprehension of immediate happenings is obvious. A comprehensive and satisfactory definition is difficult, though we all understand what the term means.

If we look upon consciousness as covering a wide field of immediate experience, we can regard attention as its focus point at which we are most intimately aware of any stimuli that fall. Awareness is concentrated here so that consciousness becomes more or less concerned with one thing only at a time to the exclusion of other stimuli, unless these make a more potent or urgent call on it.

Attention may, in the first place, be held by anything which excites interest, by either a happening in the external world or by a series of thoughts or ideas, as when we inspect a picture or read a book. But it is also, to some extent, under the control of will, and can be directed by voluntary effort to anything of interest or importance. This voluntary direction or focusing of attention is often spoken of as concentration. It determines greater efficiency in any physical or mental task that is undertaken, and more accurate performance. Attention tends, however, to fluctuate, and an effort is necessary to keep it fixed on its object. Failure to maintain it adequately is a common symptom in the psychoneuroses, but it occurs also in acute physical diseases, in diffuse affections of the brain and in states of exhaustion.

Orientation.—While inability of a conscious patient to recognise the spatial relations of objects to one another or to self may result from local disease of the brain (p. 155), failure to appreciate immediate surroundings or the place or situation in which he is at the moment, and disorientation in time, are primarily psychogenic disorders, though frequently due to organic disturbances, as trauma or the action of poisons on the brain. It may accompany or follow a period of confusion, or result from failure at the time to recognise or to remember what happened in the immediate past. More rarely it is a primary disorder; the patient does not know where he is in space or time. He may be unable to orientate himself in new surroundings or to picture to himself complicated spatial relations previously known.

Suggestibility is a state in which ideas or trains of thought may readily be influenced by external or internal agents, or by the statements or conduct of another person. Even normal persons are suggestible; anyone can walk along a plank lying on firm ground, but may be unable to do so when it spans an abyss. Suggestibility is particularly potent in periods of stress, emotional tension, mental exhaustion and in physical ill-health. In susceptible persons it may disorder even perception, especially when the object perceived is vague or indefinite; a shadow may be accepted as a spectre, an ordinary happening may become a transcendental manifestation, and phantasies suggested under suitable conditions may be confused in memory with actual events. It plays a large part in emotional life, and particularly in the sex sphere.

Abnormal suggestibility is the essential basis of many of the palsies, spasms and other physical symptoms of hysteria, the essential nature of which is conversion of an idea into symptoms. These may be suggested

N*

from without, as by observation of a similar disorder in another person, and even by clinical examination; or they may result from auto-suggestion, an injury to a limb being followed by loss of power, a laryngitis by aphonia, a temporary weakness or numbness by a psychogenic palsy or anæsthesia.

The importance of suggestion in clinical medicine, and particularly in neurology, is twofold: in the first place, it may be the origin of symptoms; and, in the second, the most effective agent in their removal. It must also be remembered that there is always a risk of suggesting to susceptible persons symptoms not previously existent, and of obtaining an inaccurate history by leading questions or inexpert cross-examination.

APPENDIX

A Scheme for the Clinical Investigation of the Functions of the Nervous System

THE advantage of employing a standard method or scheme in the examination of a patient who presents, or may present, signs of disorder in the functions of the nervous system is that it assures an adequate investigation in the shortest possible time, reduces the risk of oversight or omission of symptoms and enables the clinician to arrange his observations in a concise and logical manner. Frequently such a scheme can serve only as a preliminary or general survey of a case; facts brought to light by it, or special disorders, may require fuller investigation or the use of additional methods.

The aim of any scheme or plan of operation should be to ensure a methodical investigation of the separate functions of the nervous system; the use of the simplest methods that can furnish reliable results or observations, and the arrangement of tests so that the analysis or interpretation of each observation should be, as far as possible, independent of facts revealed by subsequent tests should be adopted, though a final conclusion can be reached only by correlation of all available evidence.

Many schemes are in use: the following will prove adequate for a preliminary examination of most cases. It may, however, be necessary or advisable to vary the sequence of tests, or modify them according to the state of the patient or the nature of his illness.

Special Senses

Smell.—Exclude local conditions as rhinitis, catarrh, etc. Use standard set of common odours, as camphor, cloves, peppermint, asafœtida.

Taste.—Apply the terminals of a torch battery to each side of the tongue.

Vision.—*Acuity of Central Vision* after errors of refraction have been corrected and opacities and other abnormalities of the media have been allowed for. Extent of *visual fields* for white and colours, first by confrontation methods and later, if necessary, by use of a perimeter. Presence or absence of *scotomata*, or areas of defective vision within the fields, first by confrontation and later by use of a perimeter or a Bjerrum's screen. *Ophthalmoscopic examination*, noting the edges and central pit of each optic disc, the colour of each disc, the condition of the retinæ, particularly of the macular regions, and the state of the retinal vessels.

Hearing.—Response to whispered voice, to a watch or tuning-fork. Conduction of sound of a vibrating tuning-fork through air and through bone. Lateralisation of sound of tuning-fork placed on middle line of skull. Presence of tinnitus.

CRANIAL NERVES

Third, Fourth and Sixth Nerves.—Range of movements of each eye and of conjugate movements. Presence or absence of squint, diplopia or nystagmus. Size, symmetry and regularity of pupils. Direct and consensual reaction of the pupils to light and on convergence. Posture and movement of the lids.

Fifth Nerve.—Size of the masseter and temporal muscles when contracted. Deviation of lower jaw on opening and closing the mouth, preferably against resistance. Sensibility of the face to touch, pin-prick and temperature. Corneal reflexes.

Seventh Nerve.—Expression and symmetry of face at rest. Voluntary and expressional movements of the upper and lower portions of the face.

Ninth and Tenth Nerves.—Position and movement of the soft palate. Palatal and pharyngeal reflexes. Position and movements of the vocal cords as seen by the laryngoscope. Articulation, phonation and swallowing.

Twelth Nerve.—Presence or absence of wasting, fibrillation and tremor of the tongue. Movements of the tongue.

MOTOR SYSTEM

Presence of atrophy or fisciculation of muscles. Tone of muscles; nature of increase of tone if present. Power of contraction of individual muscles (in peripheral lesions) and strength of movement of each segment of the limbs and of the trunk. Automatic movements, as swinging the arms in walking. Co-ordination of movement, testing first simple, later more complicated movements, as gait and the use of tools. Influence of excluding vision on accuracy of movement. Alternating movements. Presence or absence of involuntary movements.

REFLEXES

Note presence, absence or modification of the following:—

Tendon Jerks.—Flexion and extension reflexes of the forearm and finger-jerks. Knee and ankle jerks.

Superficial or Cutaneous Reflexes.—Abdominal, cremasteric and plantar reflexes.

SENSATION

Spontaneous Sensations.—Presence or absence of pain and abnormal sensations. Their nature, distribution and the factors that influence them if present.

Cutaneous Sensibility.—Response to tactile, painful and thermal stimuli. Localisation of stimuli and discrimination of compass points.

Proprioceptive Sensibility.—Postural sensation. Influence of excluding vision when standing erect. Recognition of the size, shape, form and weight of objects. Identification of familiar objects and tissues by handling. Appreciation of vibration. Pain on pressure of subcutaneous structures.

BLADDER AND RECTUM

Presence of difficulty in starting, or urgency of micturition. Tendency to incontinence, either massive or dribbling, and sensation of escape of urine. Complete emptying of bladder. Anal control, especially after taking purgatives. Anal reflex.

ENQUIRY INTO SEXUAL FUNCTIONS

MENTAL STATE

State of consciousness. Mood and emotional reactions. Memory for recent and remote events. Attention. Orientation in time and place. Hallucinations, delusions or change in conduct.

SPEECH

See tests for Aphasia, p. 147.

INDEX

185

PRINTED BY NEILL AND CO. LTD., EDINBURGH